Menopause

A Natural and Spiritual Journey

Colette Brown

AYNI
BOOKS

Winchester, UK
Washington, USA

First published by Ayni Books, 2012
Ayni Books is an imprint of John Hunt Publishing Ltd., Laurel House, Station Approach,
Alresford, Hants, SO24 9JH, UK
office1@o-books.net
www.o-books.com

For distributor details and how to order please visit the 'Ordering' section on our website.

Text copyright: Colette Brown 2011

ISBN: 978 1 78099 046 0

A CIP catalogue record for this book is available from the British Library.

Design: Lee Nash

Printed and bound by CPI Group (UK) Ltd, Croydon, CR0 4YY
Printed in the USA by Offset Paperback Mfrs, Inc

We operate a distinctive and ethical publishing philosophy in all
areas of our business, from our global network of authors to
production and worldwide distribution.

CONTENTS

For Sooz: my spirit sister, my accomplice!
For Jennifer and Jillian, my reasons for being.

Introduction

There are many books on the market that are focused on physical menopause symptoms and how to control them. There are others that are more focused on the emotional and mental symptoms that can emerge at this great time of change. These books are helpful and can lead to a greater understanding of the process. But my menopause was, to me, first and foremost a spiritual journey, a time of change in spiritual outlook and a time where I needed to understand more about this new place of 'moon pause'.

As I began to experience physical and mental symptoms, my spiritual beliefs seemed to be changing and I felt out of sorts with my previous beliefs and life patterns. This in turn seemed to aggravate the emotional fragility I was feeling and the mood swings.

I have long felt that my spirituality was intrinsic in my life outlook and my persona. To feel this shift and not to have an understanding of 'why?' left me bereft. I felt I was no longer strong, no longer in control of my spiritual life and therefore no longer in control of my emotions or my mental state. I knew I had to take a journey into the links between my spirituality and menopause and all the resulting highs and lows that were bound to follow. What made this more necessary was that I felt I needed this information to help other sisters and friends. In my life, my little spiritual circle was full of younger women who looked to me for spiritual advice and guidance. I follow a natural, shamanic path and as such, wished my menopause to be natural and as spiritual a journey as possible. I felt a responsibility and the need to monitor my feelings and find a way that menopause could be interpreted spiritually. If I was to be the first 'grandmother' or 'wise woman' in my circle, then I had to make sure I had answers for those that entered this change after me. I needed to be unselfish and to see this as finding a path that could be followed by younger women when their time came.

So, I began to do daily meditations on how I was feeling spiritually and take note of how I was also feeling emotionally, mentally and physically. Sometimes this was the other way round with e.g. a physical symptom leading the way. This proved very beneficial in helping go forward on days when my belief in myself was challenged and also when symptoms became almost too much to bear. I also identified some major hurdles spiritually and also some very worrying emotional aspects. For these I created individual meditations and healing mantras. Spiritually, I felt ungrounded, lost and very insecure. Emotionally I felt jaded, irritable and very, very fragile. But the mental mood swings were the worst. I was like Scottish weather...four seasons in one day. I could be perfectly happy one minute and in the depth of despair the next. My husband and children never knew when the next flood of tears would happen. From being a relatively calm and placid person, I found I had a temper and a tongue to match it. I have always had a wee soft spot for myself, prided myself on being a nice person with heaps of compassion and lots of patience for others. This 'me' seemed to be going and the new me wasn't someone I liked. I knew I had to do something and it had to begin with my spirituality which defines me. I knew I wanted a natural menopause with no HRT, antidepressants or sedatives, all of which were offered by my very caring doctor who joked when I asked if 'I truly was going through menopause?' he answered with a grin ' with all the symptoms you have , you ARE menopause!!'. My doctor was helpful and supportive and he never forced medicines on me. He offered them and then took my 'no' answer as a basis for seeing what else could be done to be helpful. He left the door open for me if I changed my mind about pharmaceutical help and was always content to let me 'wait and see'. Many women are not so lucky.

I was going to have to depend on *me* and to find a way through

2

this natural change of life in a way that made it a journey of hope and acceptance. It hasn't been easy and my way may well not suit you. There is nothing wrong with having some medical help. In fact some symptoms of menopause do need professional help and it would be unwise to ignore professional guidance e.g. where bone density is concerned. This book is more aimed at someone who has no great underlying problems physically, mentally or emotionally as they head towards menopause. It is for women who feel that they want to explore the spiritual journey alongside the more tangible journey. It is for those who want to explore the complexity of how spirituality, emotions and thought all affect the physical and how all need to be in balance and in harmony, if the journey is to be in any way beneficial and the outcome, serene. I chose to make this journey without the aid of herbal medicines as well. This was mainly to see if it could be done with simply nothing but meditation and spiritual awareness. If I had introduced an herbal remedy I would not have been truly sure what aspect was having a beneficial effect. Plus not all herbal remedies are efficacious and some can be quite toxic if taken in the wrong dose. Always consult your herbalist or pharmacist before taking herbal remedies.

The following chapters explore how to be in balance through the day to day changes of the body, mind and soul. Some are general and some are based on particular issues that many moon pause women go through e.g. body image, self belief, mental fog, lack of libido etc etc. Follow me through my journey, do the meditations, repeat the mantras as necessary and honor yourself by giving time and energy to the process. This is YOUR time. It is YOUR journey. It is better to be in control of it as much as possible, to feel that it is your right to explore yourself and your feelings. Gift yourself this time of understanding and make it the best it can be for YOU.

The meditations in each chapter can be done after reading my experiences and can be adapted to suit your own belief system.

You will need to find your 'sacred space' first: the place where you can be alone and not be disturbed. It is better to say the mantras out loud or chant them initially. Then you can say them into yourself in places where saying them out loud or bursting into a chant might be inappropriate e.g. workplace. Repetition is the key. Use your own words if you can. Mine are just a guide, words that suited me and I was familiar with. I use the term 'Grandmother ' to symbolise the wise woman phase of spirituality. Some spiritualities say 'crone' but I still have problems with the word because when I was a child we used it to signify an old woman who was ugly, bedraggled and a bit odd and crazy, like the old witch in Walt Disney's Snow White. Its connotations don't inspire me the way 'grandmother' or 'wise woman' do. This is truly personal so use whatever word you feel comfortable with. I also use the word 'Spirit' in meditation and mantras to mean Great Spirit, the connection between all things, the energy of life and the Universe. You may prefer to connect with a particular goddess or deity that is important to you. In some meditations I have indeed felt drawn to a particular goddess but in general, I have given up my intent to Spirit.

Remember to do what suits you. It is your personal journey.

I also use certain crystals during meditations that help with individual energy sought or just for the focus they bring. Crystals can be bought from any good Body, Mind and Soul shop and also on the internet. My little bag contains moonstone, blood stone, citrine, fluorite, hematite, selenite, amethyst, aquamarine, green calcite, and sodalite. Feel the energy from each crystal and enjoy learning its power. Hold the crystal in your palm and cup your other palm over it. Let the energy pulsate into you and out of you again. Some crystals energise, others ground you and others take in negativity.

Make sure that you allow at least 30 minutes for each meditation and try to do them once a day. Use the general one for 'everyday' days and the more specific ones for specific problems or feelings. Wear loose, comfortable, layered clothing and have a wee blanket in case you feel cold. Light an appropriate candle or incense and have some drinking water beside you. Even if the meditations don't come easy at first, familiarity will bring greater connection. And in the worst case scenario that you have just sat still for half an hour and not been hassled by partners or teenagers, then that to me is a good outcome too! Keep a notepad and pen beside you to jot down any thoughts or insights that come up. This will help you modify and progress to further meditations. And if you don't manage the meditations and mantras then at least you may enjoy reading of my personal experiences. These will show that you are not alone or going mad. Good luck!

Chapter One

Early Days

I have always had problems with my menstruation or moon flow. I took my first 'moon' or period on the stroke of midnight on New Year's Eve when I was eleven. What followed was adolescent years of pain and heavy periods, anaemia and faints. My mum encouraged me by saying that the earlier you started your periods, the longer you went before menopause, which protected your bones and helped you feel young. She actually didn't have this experience herself as she had a radical hysterectomy when she was forty right after I was born by caesarean section. So I never really knew at what age I would go through it based on hereditary factors but I felt I would be in my mid fifties anyway.

I had three very easy conceptions and had no fertility problems although I suffered from severe pains due to endometriosis in my forties. I also had to have two D and C's to remove a polyp and some fibroids. By age 47 I had been through so many gynae investigations that I was sick and tired of being poked and prodded and actually felt that when the time came, I would welcome menopause with open arms. I still thought it would be about age 55 though. On a few occasions it had been suggested that a hysterectomy might be a good course of action. But I felt spiritually connected to my womb. I have participated in a few Native American moon sweat lodges (sweat lodges only for women) and had even set up a moon lodge for monthly prayers and meditations with some close spiritual women friends. As a professional clairvoyant, I knew that I felt things through my womb and whether or not this was right, I didn't want to lose it. When asked by some consultants why I wanted to persevere with medication to cut blood loss etc, my answer of 'I have a spiritual connection to my uterus' was met by blank faces. But on one occasion I was seen by a wonderful Chinese woman consultant who replied with 'well, let's see how we can manage your condition then'. Of course, any sinister disease had been ruled out. I was in no danger.

So I soldiered on and after the polyp and fibroid removal expected things to be a bit better. It was for a while but then I developed very heavy periods and had such bad pain that I returned to see my local doctor. He said that it might be the countdown to menopause and that we would manage the pain with medication and wait and see what happened. He referred me back to the hospital for a further scan which proved to be clear. For the next 4 months I bled every 2 weeks and became very tired and low. Then suddenly...nothing! I missed a period and thought little of it as I was sure that my body was just adjusting to all the after effects of the last year. Then came the terrible mood swings, the tiredness and loss of libido. At the same time I felt emotionally drained and short of my usual sparkle. But I struggled on and tried to keep on a happy face. My doctor confirmed I was in menopause and I decided just to get on with it.

But then I noticed something more sinister. I wasn't concentrating on my prayers or meditations the way I used to. I work as a clairvoyant tarot reader and am quite disciplined in making sure I meditate and 'open up' for at least an hour before I do a reading. The hour would go by and I would have lost the place in my opening prayers and intents for the reading. I felt bad about this and kept restarting them and apologising to the Universe for not being in the zone. The readings didn't suffer so I felt the universe was forgiving or more understanding of my time in life than I was. I was unhappy with my observance of my path and had no energy to change it. I felt I may lose my gift or in some way let people down. I was insecure in my spirituality and this had never happened to me in 14 years since starting to follow a shamanic path. This hit me hard. But it was like a vicious circle...I had no energy to put into my path and therefore I was getting no energy or real connection back. And the more I lost my way spiritually, the more I went downhill emotionally and mentally. It was time to get back to basics and find out where I stood spiritually. This was the key that would help me, I was sure, find the energy to pull myself out of what was fast resembling a deep pit of tiredness and demotivation.

So I went back to the basic teachings of the Medicine Wheel. There are many differing examples of Medicine Wheels which vary between tribes. Some have different associations with the directions and energies and elements. My advice if using the Medicine Wheel is to find one that resonates with you and stick with it. Or you can use the one below which is a relatively common one. In the Native American Medicine Wheel there are primarily four directions all associated with many things but firstly based on the four aspects of life we need to keep in balance i.e. spirituality, the emotions, the physical and the intellect. For the centre or soul to be in harmony, or complete, all these directions must be kept in balance as much as possible. This is a very, very simplistic explanation but is all that is needed now to understand where I am coming from. In the east direction sits the place of spirituality, in the south, the emotions, the west represents the physical and the north is where the intellect resides. It is important to balance across each axis first. In looking at this it confirmed what I felt: that my spirituality was being affected by my physical problems and vice versa. (See diagram 1, overleaf)

Before you start the first meditation, let me show you the two ways of approaching how to understand where the imbalances are on a day to day basis. Firstly, familiarize yourself with the four directions of the Medicine Wheel and what attributes they have i.e. east equals spirituality, south equals emotions, west equals physical and the north equals intellect. The centre of the

Medicine Wheel

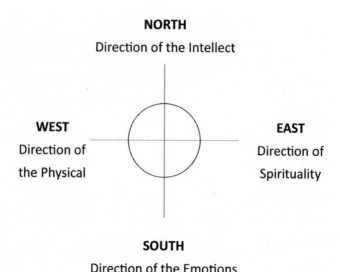

NORTH

Direction of the Intellect

WEST

Direction of
the Physical

EAST

Direction of
Spirituality

SOUTH

Direction of the Emotions

wheel is the soul. To have the soul in balance, all the directions must be in harmony. If you read the tarot, oracle cards or any other form of inspirational cards, then shuffle them and cut them. Place the first card in the east and then follow clockwise around the directions, placing the fifth card in the centre or soul position. Look at the cards and see what they tell you about how you are in each direction at that time. If a negative card is in one direction, work on that in your meditation and develop a mantra for it. If you have two negative cards placed in directions, work on both etc. If you have negative cards in all directions..........take action...you are well out of sorts! If the card that falls in the centre or soul position is positive, then this will help you go forward in a good and upbeat way. But if it is negative, your soul is struggling and it is even more important to give yourself meditation time and maybe solitude on that day. By doing a daily Medicine Wheel spread you can keep an eye on your progress.

If you do not have any divination cards, then simply ask yourself how you feel in each direction, note positive or negative and work on it. It will be harder to judge the feeling of the centre or soul, so maybe just focus on the directions if you don't use cards. You may benefit from placing a symbol in each direction. Our brains have been shown to connect with symbols better than words. So maybe place personal symbol that connects you to spirituality e.g. a cross, an amulet, a rune stone in the east direction. In the south, place something that represents the emotions e.g. a heart shaped crystal, a family photo. In the west, use a symbol of the physical. This could be a drawing of a body or a piece of hair. In the north, you could put a symbol of intellect e.g. a book or a graduation photo.

The first meditation:

This will be general and based on what your Medicine Wheel investigation tells you. Try to do it daily but use another more specific one (from further chapters) if you are feeling a more specific problem e.g. crisis of confidence or 'empty nest'. These specific ones follow in subsequent chapters.

Crystals:

Moonstone. This will help you connect with your moon flow or lack of it. It allows the gentle energy of the moon to connect with you and calm you.

Fluorite, to help you open up spiritually and sense your true feelings.

How do I really feel?

(I am worried and all out of sorts. I feel so stressed and so upset that what I have felt spiritually has become mundane and has lost its delight for me. I am angry and sad that I seem to have lost my way. My spirituality is so much a part of me and if I am losing this, then I am losing myself. I feel tired and weepy and not very attractive just now. My brain doesn't want to cope with the problems of life and I feel like running away. I am irritable and unhappy and can't seem to empathize with people the way I have in the past. Oh, Spirit, I am confused and low. What can I do? What is really wrong? Am I ill? Am I depressed? And if so, what have I to be depressed about? My life is fine. I have many blessings. I have love in my life. I feel ungrateful and self centred and it hurts to feel this way. Help me, Spirit to understand this process of moon pause. Let me accept it and move through it in a good and honourable way. Let me learn from it and become all I can be. Let me not be diminished by it. Help me Spirit to see the spiritual path unfolding before me. Help me to work through the symptoms of this menopause and to cut myself some slack as I do it. I am not perfect. I am human and I am going through a part of human life. It is natural. It is my time. Guide me.)

What can I do today to help me?
(I can let myself off the hook for how emotional I am feeling. I can give what I have to give and accept there is a limit on this for the moment. I can give myself some time to think about things and I can try to accept these changes with a good heart. I can accept that I am now on the journey to being the grandmother, even if it feels premature.)

Mantra:
(I accept this journey towards moon pause. I am blessed to be here.
I accept this journey towards the Grandmother. I am blessed to have made it this far.)

Chapter 2

From Spring to Autumn

My spiritual journey has been long and varied. But I have always been intensely connected to my sixth sense or my psychic nature. Even as a young child I could see and hear spirits and had the power to predict. I had an 'imaginary ' friend who was a little Native America boy. I called him 'Nindian' as I knew he was the like the 'cowboysanindians' I watched on TV with my dad on a Saturday afternoon. He was my friend, my playmate. My 'Indian boy' grew up alongside me and eventually I recognized him as my spirit guide. My family were Roman Catholic and I had the usual ceremonies like my first Holy Communion. I loved the ceremonies and felt very connected with being 'holy'. As a teenager I attended an all girl's Catholic school and would sit in contemplation in the convent chapel. At one point I felt such a strong connection to the Virgin Mary that I wanted to be a nun. I sought out solitude as it helped me think and gave me feelings of wellbeing. I was really just meditating naturally in a quiet and spiritual environment. By the time I left school I had already delved into Judaism, Russian Orthodox religion and Buddhism. I searched spiritually for something although I did not know what I was looking for. I had posters of Jonathan Livingstone Seagull mixed in with Starsky and Hutch! At university I did the odd palm reading, but generally became caught up in Catholicism again as I prepared to be married and wanted a spiritual ceremony. In my mid twenties, the tarot found me and I became totally committed and caught up in the archetypes of the Major Arcana. The tarot made me feel complete. My spirituality was the Tarot. But the symbolism and need to explore led me towards a more earthy spirituality. I studied Norse ways and

Arthurian legends while still keeping one foot in the organised religion camp. I started to do tarot readings and my guide was with me all the way. I didn't really honour his path. He was just my friend, my guide, my one time playmate. But in 1997 I met a Native American elder and had my first experience of a sweat lodge. But before I could enter the sweatlodge, there had to be lessons, time spent understanding the Medicine Wheel teachings. As the old man explained in a gruff voice the magic of the teachings, I realised that, somewhere deep inside, I already knew them. I had lived them at one point. Maybe it was in a past life or in dream time with my spirit guide. But I knew them! From that point on, I knew exactly what path I should be on. I learned as much as I could and honored each teacher and guide who came my way. I tried to walk my talk...to walk in beauty, balance and harmony... to walk the Wheel. I did sweat lodges, a vision quest and tried to work Native American ceremonies into my life in Scotland. Not easy, but I don't feel you have to be Norse to follow a Norse path or Indian to follow a Hindu path. The same stands for Native American spirituality. Bit by bit I realized that my path was one of a shaman, based on a natural connection with the spirits of all things in this life and beyond. I was happy and contented.

When my physical menopause symptoms began to hit, it was a time of shock really as I didn't feel old enough to be menopausal. Just a generation ago, menopausal women looked old. They had thinning hair set in perms, wrinkles and wore shapeless coats. Well they did in Scotland in the nineteen sixties anyway. They were recognised for what they were; no longer fertile and heading towards old age. In a way I believe this may have made things easier. You are how you look. You are not expected to be something you are not. But my generation looks different. It is healthier, stronger and we live longer and more active lives now. So when I started menopause, it was quite a shock. I preferred mad, colorful leggings to dresses. I kept my hair long and messy. I loved make up and scent and liked the films my daughters watched and even much of their music. The chasm of the generation gap that I had with my mum simply wasn't there. My sense of self was young, fun and hippily hip! It did not match up at all with the old sense of a menopausal woman.

In my spiritual life I still felt I was in the 'mother ' time. Grandmother time was far away yet. I could ignore the potential responsibilities for a while yet. I did not feel either wise enough or committed enough to take up the role of the grandmother. Yet things were changing. In my clairvoyant consultancy, I could feel a shift. I was seeing more and more young women in their twenties and thirties. I had always connected with this age group as comrades, sharing the odd joke and seeing myself as one of them. But I began to see that this age group was approaching me in a different way. They came more with a sense of reverence or respect and I found it quite unsettling. I found myself bit by bit relating to them in a different way, giving advice in a more direct and compassionate way. They told me things like I was a confidant, a person they could trust, not someone just equal in experience. Before long it was even more obvious that they saw my older woman peering over her glasses with some strands of silver hair as someone who merited their honesty. My advice was accepted easier. I looked as though I had life experience. My age was very much working in my favour as I assumed authority and people generally listened more.

But I still did not see myself as others seemed to. I was busy and knew what I did helped many people. In my head, my mental image of a grandmother was of an old lady, with white hair, sparkly eyes, wrinkles and depth of intuition and spiritual knowledge of great magnitude...something to aspire to but not quite yet! A bit like 'God, please make me good...but not yet!

So there was a gulf between where I was physically and what I felt like spiritually, and my perception of what a grandmother

or wise woman looked like and her spiritual powers and responsibilities. It was time to return to the Medicine Wheel.

The Medicine Wheel also reflects the seasons and the seasons
of life. See diagram 2.

Medicine Wheel

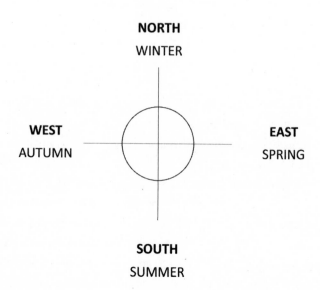

NORTH
WINTER

WEST
AUTUMN

EAST
SPRING

SOUTH
SUMMER

The four quadrants represent different times in our lives.
North to east is birth through to adolescence. East to south is the
place of growing maturity, of menstruation and of preparing to
mother. South to west is the place of mature mothering and
connecting more with our families. West to north, of heading
towards death and connecting with the ancestors. The east
direction represents spring; the south, summer; the west, autumn
and the north , winter. Menopause is right on the cusp between
the third and fourth quadrant. It bridges the gap between mother
and grandmother. It is a special place. It is where every physical
symptom and spiritual movement was telling me I was. I had just

better get used to it!

There was also the problem with my name. Many years ago I had been gifted the spirit name 'Quiets the Storm'. It was a name that was full of honor and responsibility. It was seen as a name that showed that I was caring and compassionate and that I 'quietened other peoples' storms or troubles. It always linked me to weather prediction, to the tribal people who understood weather and when to move camp etc when winter was coming. I liked this name! Its 'stormy' side suited my hair, my impulsive nature and my love of standing outside in thunder storms. Also, after many years of calling my guide 'Nindian' or my Native American guide, he had finally told me after I was gifted this name, that his name was White Storm. Another 'storm' name which I felt linked us even more. But during a deep meditation, White Storm called me 'Grandmother Sunfire'. It panicked me. That wasn't me. I was a storm name. I connected to the moon. I wasn't a sun person. I loved the connection to my guide's name. Would he now leave me? But I talked this new name over with an Apache elder who explained that it was a very good name indeed and that I should work with it, to discover what it really meant to me. These meditations on my new name were incredibly personal and in depth and I choose to keep them that way. The outcome was that I came to understand that my 'feeling' centre was moving from my womb to my heart and that the creative fire within me was about to be unleashed.

Meditation: for spiritual clarity

Crystals:
Selenite for connection to higher beings and sodalite to help
    understand the truth of the spiritual path.

How do I really feel now?
(Aho Great Spirit, I come to you in honor and respect. I come on the bridge between Mother and Grandmother and I come asking

for insight into my new role and into my way forward. Can you reassure me that I am ready for this transition? Can you give me a sign? I am fearful of the responsibility of being a wise woman, of being the person who advises the younger women and nurtures them. I am scared of the responsibility of being the person who sees the bigger picture. Yet, I long to truly be that person. I feel that I could honor that role. I know by the way younger woman come to me that they seek wisdom from me. They see me as mature and mystical. Help me se myself through their eyes. Help me step up and be ready as best I can to honor Grandmother Sunfire, to be a wisdom keeper. As I cross the bridge into the fourth quadrant, let me explore my needs and the needs of my greater community.)

What can I do to help myself now?
(I can make sure that I meditate every day on this bridge. I can seek out elders and other moonpause women to hear their stories and to draw strength from their presence. I can become familiar with my new name and all that it holds. A name is power and this indeed is a powerful name. I can spend time being alone and contemplating my community, the earth and her needs. I can walk with dignity and teach by example so that the young women know that they are supported.)

Mantra:
(Spirit. Let me honor my new name. I am on my way to being
   Grandmother Sunfire!
Akehela! Mitakuye Oyasin!)

Chapter 3

Crisis of Confidence

My parents had brought me up to be confident and know my self worth. They were older parents and were mellower by the time I came along. I wasn't a well child and attended a lot of hospitals due to being born early and having some problems. As a result of German Measles when I was three I was hard of hearing and needed glasses for a bad squint. My palate and nose hadn't developed properly and I needed facial surgery and corrective dentistry. And the kind Creator added ginger hair and freckles to this mix! I was a child just waiting to be bullied. But my mum and my dad adored me and told me I was wonderful and beautiful and special. I grew up feeling appreciated and well loved. I had good friends, went to an all girl's school that rewarded hard work and ability and generally believed that I could achieve whatever I wanted. I was presented to the Queen and Prince Charles for community work in my teens. I achieved a decent honors degree and went on to do well in my career in pharmacy. Even when I gave pharmacy up to become a full time clairvoyant, I did it with confidence and a sense that I could achieve my hopes and dreams. My career as a clairvoyant and columnist has been good and I never felt out of place when reading for celebrities or business whiz kids. I even did TV and radio.

So, when moon pause started I was shocked to feel this confidence slip away and be replaced by self doubt and negative self awareness. There were times when I just said No right away to things I would have jumped at before. I felt that I would mess up or not show myself off to my best. Granted, this also coincided with having to wear a second hearing device as my hearing was deteriorating too. I am sure this didn't help. Being in a room with people with a noisy background was terrifying and I wouldn't do an 'event' without my husband or daughter accompanying me.

I couldn't understand why, when I was once so confident, that now I was scared and wanted to be invisible and left alone. It was easier to be just getting on with work and be safe within my self set limitations. But this had never been my way before. The physical symptoms of sweats and red, flushed cheeks didn't help. How can you appear confident when you look like you are nervous and having a panic attack? How can you feel confidence in yourself when your carefully applied make up has just slid off and your hair is limp and your lovely dress is feeling like wet Clingfilm? It was very hard to keep an ounce of confidence and self belief.

Yet my spirituality had always given me confidence too. It taught me how to keep in balance and to walk in harmony with my inner self and my body. So why was this not helping now? I tried to think of myself as a goddess, as the epitome of womanhood. These were standard symptoms weren't they? I am Everywoman and Everywoman is me. Therefore, get a grip and just do it. That didn't work. It just made me less confident in myself as woman and less connected to the universal 'goddess'. So back to the meditations and mantras. This would need to be a powerful one as it was a truly important issue. How could I expect the people who came to me for advice to believe in what I said if I was coming over lacking in confidence and self worth?

Meditation: for lack of confidence
Crystals:
Citrine, for happy bright confident feelings and green calcite to
    ground these feelings and bring a sense of self worth.

What do I really feel?
(Oh Spirit, my confidence has gone. My faith in myself has gone.

I feel weak and panicky and not at all able to take on the roles I used to do without thinking about them. I feel I am letting myself down and others. The confidence my parents inspired in me is no longer there. My family still tell me I am good at what I do and I am complimented on my work. But I feel out of sorts, adolescent and I do not believe in myself any more. I have lost confidence in my spirituality to guide me through as it has done many times before. I am worried that this will be self fulfilling and I will lose who I am and my sense of being connected to the Great Spirit. Help me.)

What can I do today to help me?
(I can look at what I have achieved. I can see that people don't really perceive me as different to before. I can see the love for me. I can make time to do the physical things that will help me regain my confidence in my body, mind and soul. I can just say yes to things rather than hiding from potential disasters. I can realize that I am whole and good and that I can achieve all that I want to in life. I can believe that this phase will end with me being more spiritually aware, not less.)

Mantra:
(I believe in myself as a woman, partner, mother, sister, friend and co-worker.
I am as good as the next person and WILL take my confidence and power back: if only for today.)

Chapter 4

Sweaty Betty, Chin Hair and Belly Hell

I played football, rode my bike and hiked for miles in hot summers as a child. I played volleyball and danced as a teenager. I loved dancing until I dropped at nights out at concerts in my twenties and thirties. In my forties I took part in over 40 Native American sweat lodges for purification and healing. I knew what sweat was! But actually, I didn't! There is another type of sweat that has no grand feelings of either physical victory or spiritual purification associated with it. This sweat is extreme, debilitating and highly embarrassing. Menopausal sweats or hot flushes redefine what it is to sweat. I don't even remember the first one as I think I must have just thought it was a reaction to the heat or something I was doing. I don't remember the second one either...but after a few I was starting to feel that something was not right. The hot flushes were there even before I had the heavy bleeds that pre-empted menopause. In fact, they may even have been my first symptom.

I remember being out shopping with my daughters and was feeling very hot. I just wanted leave but I met an old friend of the family on the way to the exit. As I was talking to her, I felt as though my face was turning the colour of a plum. Quite embarrassing! And I felt she could sense my impatience to be out of the hot shopping mall. This made me worse and I could feel myself sweating under my long curly hair. This was not a little bit of sweat though: it was pouring down my back. My forehead was soaking wet and to my discomfort, sweat was dripping onto my eyelids! Then the worst...I noticed that my blue silk top had drops of rain splashing down the front! How could it be raining in a shopping mall? My elder daughter took out a handkerchief and started to dab the ends of my hair. Then I realised that the sweat from my head and hair was actually dripping onto my top! This panicked me even more and that made the sweats worse. By this time, my top was clinging to my back, I felt light headed and thought I might faint. Excuses were made and my daughters marched me to my car. I felt worn out, embarrassed and completely soaked through! It made me wary of shopping, silk tops and hot days!

There was more to come. I could be ready for a night out and have a wee glass of wine before I went. Bad idea! Alcohol made the sweats come on with a vengeance. My make up slid off my face, I would have to change my dress, my hair would be wet and I would be grumpy and fed up and not want to go out after all. If I was in anyway in a hurry or nervous, the sweats would descend like a red torrent of hot mist. I loved cooking Sunday roast for the family and persevered. But most times when I had put everything out, I didn't feel like eating because I was so hot and bothered. A horrible side effect of the sweats was that it got under both my hearing devices and made them totally uncomfortable and blocked so I had to take them out for a while, leaving me feeling even more distressed. (Maybe that is too much information? At least I am being truly honest). I took to carrying a fresh body spray everywhere with me, loads of tissues and a cool can of coke, not to drink, but to place on my neck to cool me down! Night sweats were not as bad as daytime ones as at least there was a cool shower on hand. But my husband took to lying as far away from me as he could as I was generating enough heat to power the whole of Glasgow! Then I would become cold due to the sweat cooling and would need the duvet and then I would sweat again, starting the whole process over again.

Then, one day, as I was putting on my make up, I noticed what looked like a small blackhead on my chin. I was always careful of my skin as it had flared up with acne rosacea when I was going through my divorce due to stress. A blackhead could be the start.

But on closer inspection I was horrified: it was the tip of a course, black hair. I have pale coloring and red/blonde hair and the thought of a big black beard brought on yet another hot flush! Panic! Tweezers! Gone! Forget it. It won't come back! But it did, regularly! Sometimes the downy hair on my neck seemed a bit too downy too! There was no way I was having a beard! So every day, the tweezers came out and if there was anything that they could catch, it was plucked away. I didn't have much, just one wee black persistent one and the odd short blonde one. Many women suffer more. But it isn't so much how many, but that they are there at all. Visions of beardy old woman wrapped in shawls, with no teeth came to mind. NO!

There was also the fact that although I had lost some weight, that my waist measurement was steadily climbing. I have been over weight since my mid twenties but always had an hour glass shape. Now my waist wasn't going in and from the side I looked 8 months pregnant. This made my breasts look less becoming and also made me feel so out of proportion. I had to change the way I dressed a little. No more fitted dresses or trousers with uncomfortable waistbands.

Altogether, with the sweats, my new found chin hair and my new body shape, my body image was in meltdown! I mentioned my belly shape to my wonderful husband who, instead of saying that he hadn't noticed, said that he had ...but not to worry, it would settle once I was through menopause! His honest, caring answer made me feel worse. What he was trying to say was that it didn't matter to him, but I just 'heard' that he had noticed it. I didn't give up though. I dressed nicely, always had nice manicured nails and treated myself to nice skin care and wore my make up even if it didn't last an hour. I had found a lovely photo of me at my first wedding in 1982. It is such a lovely photo and I must admit I did look awfully pretty in it. I posted it with other family photos on Facebook. One of my male friends who had only known me about 10 years posted beside it ...'it's a shame we get old!' Thanks mate! How could I reconcile that lovely bride with the older me? Back to the spiritual before I put my head in a bag and only ever worked online forever!

Meditation: for crisis of body image

Crystals:

Amethyst, to take away negative feelings.

Aquamarine, to go with the flow and maybe help with the sweats.

How am I really feeling?

(Oh Spirit, I am feeling so different physically. In my head I still feel sixteen. but my body is older and I am feeling short changed by the changes! I don't mind the wrinkles so much. They are signs of my life on my face. But chin hair is mannish and I am not a man! It makes me feel so unattractive and scared that it will get worse. My body shape is annoying. My clothes don't fit and my breasts are droopy and my skin is blotchier due to the cursed sweats. My body confidence is low and it is affecting my sense of sexuality and my day to day life. Oh Spirit, help me to see myself as I truly am and accept what I cannot change. But let me also not give up and give me the energy to keep doing what I can to feel and look good. I am older but I am still pretty. My wit and humor are intact and I can still flirt. Let me still be sexual and happy in my own new, aging body!)

Do this meditation after you have stripped off in front of a full length mirror! It is hard but what is the worst that can happen? You will see every wrinkle, roll of fat and droop. But really, does it matter? You are still you; you are still the spiritual person, the girl/woman and now heading towards the grandmother! Respect!

Mantra:

(Spirit, my body is older and is showing the signs of physical
   decline.

But I am still the same as I ever was, just older and wiser!)

Chapter 5

Mood Swing Purgatory

I wasn't ever that moody. Maybe as an adolescent and certainly when I was older and suffered from PMT. But it was controlled by evening primrose oil capsules and more rest. I only was truly irritable if I was tired or in pain. But then I would just have some quiet time and withdraw from things a wee bit. I never suffered from post natal depression after my children's births and only once was on anti depressants. This was for two months after my dad died and I came off them quickly as I felt that they were stopping the grieving process and that it would eventually have to be lived through. They also made me sleepy and unfocused in work as a pharmacist. (This was in the mid nineties and there are better antidepressants available now with less side effects.) My first husband was clinically depressed and I saw him struggle with even daily tasks. I can honestly say I had never been so low that life seemed not worth it. Because I had lived with depression in someone I loved for the best part of 23 years, I was fully aware of what true depression is: it is not the blues, it is not 'feeling a bit low', it is crippling and desolate. Even when I felt low or sad I could still see the beauty in a flower or a child's smile. I feel if something ordinary can give you joy, you are not really depressed.

I had been very tired due to all the gynae problems I had suffered and felt that it was tiredness that had started to make me feel low and bit dejected. But when the excess bleeding had stopped and I began to feel a bit more stable physically, I was worried at the way I was feeling mentally. It wasn't as though I was low all the time. In fact I would say that most of the time I was fine. But every so often a kind of black mist would descend making me feel hopeless, sad and lacking in will power to push it away. When this happened I would just cry. The tears would spill out and just keep coming until I looked liked a red faced, swollen eyed caricature. And then, just as quickly, I would be fine and happy and saying 'Oh Dear! What was that about?' and getting on with things to hide my embarrassment. Two minutes later I would have a fit of giggles over something random my daughter had said and would be bent double with laughter, tears streaming out of my eyes again... but this time with mirth. I couldn't stop laughing sometimes at the most inappropriate moments. Once, while in a cinema with my daughters to see a film, my older daughter said something drole and away I went. It wasn't actually THAT funny but I was laughing, choking and crying as the film started with folk turning to look at me as though I was mad. So I pushed my hand in my mouth and hoped for the best. But every so often, I would have a flashback to what my daughter had said and away I would go again. It was hell but the more I tried to stop laughing and giggling the worse it was. Eventually, my daughters were glaring at me so much that I shut my eyes and tried to focus on something so bland that I missed part of the film.

A comment could make me just hit the lowest ebb and the same comment a day later could have me laughing till I cried. A photo, a piece of music, a compliment, a hug...all of these could have both reactions and either depending on the moment they hit me. This was not right. But in a way it was quite a sign to myself and others that I was seriously hormonal. It gave us all some great stories and was something I could see the funny side of. But everything was so extreme.

I had asked for the film 'Pan's Labyrinth' for a present and when I watched it I was so affected that I knew I could never watch it again. Scenes from the film came unbridled into my memory for days, weeks, months after it, causing me distress and sadness. A song on the radio could have me thinking of my family in spirit and I just lost the plot. Tears and more tears and so much sorrow. Yet a silly joke could have me laughing for weeks. It could be quite inappropriate too. My daughter fell down the hall stairs and once I had checked she was all right, I just sat on the stairs and laughed till I cried. It was pure slapstick, pure joy. Every time she looked at me like 'Oh mum. That was sore. Why are you laughing?' her disapproval made it go on even longer. Eventually she was laughing at ME laughing. I felt bad, but was not in control at all. My second husband cut off his ponytail after 30 years of having one and I just couldn't stop laughing even though I thought it was nice and suited him. I am sure he thought I was just being polite when I said it was a good new look (and then ran upstairs to cry with laughter)

There seemed nothing I could do to stop these mad mood swings that caught me off guard almost every day as time went on. I did cry a lot. I laughed a lot too. And mostly I did both at the same time.

I was also becoming more and more irritable. I have never been that house-proud, but the children leaving things at their backsides began to annoy me more and more. I seemed to be mislaying things and was annoyed at myself for the extra time this added onto an already stressful day, I was angry at small things and I don't do anger well. I see it as a destructive emotion unless it can lead to a change for the better. My calls for family meetings were met with looks of 'oh here we go again...mum wants to tell us off about something!' I felt over burdened and so very close to the edge. (It is interesting that my elder daughter in reading this so far has said that 'It wasn't as bad as all that'. But I felt it was and at that point, that was all I could see.) I felt because I had been a placid person more prone to talking rather than yelling, that I was way over the line. Basically, what I felt was bad behaviour wasn't really BUT it felt that way to me.

I was so glad that these mood swings didn't ever hit while I was giving a tarot consultation. Readings can be intense and sometimes funny too but I prided myself on never being too over the top or familiar and thank the gods, this was still working. So I thought...why? Why do the mood swings not hit in these times when I am dealing with emotions and also sometimes hearing some very sad stories of peoples' lives? The only thing different was that I meditated for an hour before readings. Again, another clear link that my spirituality could help with the mad symptoms of menopause. I had realized this with the physical symptoms, but it was a great insight when I realized it could help with the mental symptoms too. The intellect is on the same axis as the emotional on The Medicine Wheel (see diagram 1). So if I could modify my thought processes a bit, then surely I could modify my emotional response too? And I felt that again meditation was the starting place to modify my thought processes.

Meditation: for mood swings
Crystals:
Moonstone, to balance out hormonal swings.
Sodalite, to help define what is really causing the mood swings from an emotional point of view.

What do I really feel?
(Oh Spirit: I am tired of being so emotionally unbalanced. I am tired of feeling so out of sorts within my day to day life. I am embarrassed by these outbursts of emotions linked to my mood swings. I feel the need to be more in balance mentally. My mood swings frighten me. I feel I am going mad at times. Please help me to bring these mood swings into balance. Help me to be less irritable and judgemental. Please let me be more generally calm and in harmony. Let me cry when I need to and laugh when I need to, but in these circumstances, let me be in control of how my moods emerge. Give me the power and confidence to accept this but also to be more in control.)

What can I do today to help me?
(I can resolve to do mini meditations throughout the day. Before a stressful event, I can allow myself time to breathe and time to relax. I can accept not only the mood swings but also that I can have a degree of control over them. I can choose the way I will react. I will monitor these moods and see what brings them on and I will be prepared for them. I can choose my response from a new list of emotions. I can feel sad without copious tears. I can feel laughter without pulling a muscle. I can be irritable without anger. I now resolve to start and finish the day with meditation and prayer.)

Mantra:
(Mood, I welcome you. Emotion, I welcome you. I will breathe through you.
I have control. I have power over this.)

Chapter 6

And Where Is My Brain?

I have an honours degree and a professional qualification. I can be a bit dizzy at times and feel I don't have much general knowledge. I know the things that I have studied and have quite a quick brain that can work laterally and see patterns in things which has been useful both in specializing in pharmacology and also in reading the tarot. I simply adore word search puzzles (but abhor crossword puzzles!) and I am good at counting and working through lists. I am not stupid. So why, in certain areas of life did my brain develop a thick fog when menopause hit? I could still see patterns in the tarot cards I so loved. I could still do word puzzles and I could add up with the best of them. However, parking a car became a nightmare. Reverse parking simply didn't work anymore and I would end up at a very odd angle while men in white vans laughed their heads off...or worse! On one occasion I simply handed my car keys to my big brother after trying to reverse out of a small driveway and let him do it for me. Total embarrassment!

If I ventured out to the shops without a list, I came back minus the things I needed but with some amazing treats that I didn't. I said things without thinking that caused hilarity all round. For example, one night I wondered out loud 'why bats could fly if they didn't have feathers?' It was quickly pointed out that aeroplanes don't have feathers either. Hhhhmmm... True!

My sense of direction, never having been great, totally left me. I couldn't multitask as I always had. If I was listening to music and someone began talking, I couldn't concentrate. Recipes that were in my head now had to be written down or I would not remember them. Peoples' names became a problem. I would use the wrong PIN codes for banking or put my card in the machine the wrong way. I nearly filled the car with diesel one day although I have never had a diesel car. I had to rely on diaries, smart phone calendars and reminders for birthdays and events. And don't even talk about multi story car parks!!! My brain was in neutral. I was no longer the driver!

Meditation: for brain fog
Crystals:
Clear quartz, for clarity of thought and dynamic energy.
Hematite, for grounding and strength.

How am I really feeling now?
(Oh Spirit, why has my intellect and memory left me? I feel silly and unprofessional. I am embarrassed when I forget a friend's name or when I forget where I have parked my car. Simple tasks simply go wrong. My concentration isn't what it used to be. I am worried that I will forget something important. I worry that I will let myself down and say something totally humiliating or wrong. Please help me be more alert or less foggy. Please help me to deal with feeling not as clever as I used to be in some areas. I would value some help here!)

What can I do now to help myself?
(I can understand that hormones can cause a foggy brain. I can cut myself some slack and laugh my head off with others when I say something daft. I can be confident that this will pass and I will be able to function on a higher intellectual level once more. I can acknowledge the things I still have no problem with like my tarot readings and my memory for song lyrics from the past. I am not ill. There is nothing wrong. I am just hormonal.)

Mantra:

(Menopause stole my brain; she can keep it for a while!
It needed a holiday anyway!)

Chapter 7

Lacklustre Libido

I would say that my libido's story was pretty normal and would match up with most females. It made its slightly uncomfortable presence felt watching Marc Bolan on TV and had a wee tug by Captain Kirk of the Starship Enterprise just before my periods started. Then it was fully awakened in early teens by David Cassidy pouting from my bedroom walls. It grew quite rabid with some rockers in the late seventies, only to become calmer and more sensual with some jazz funk in the eighties. Then it died a death after my first child was born, had a wee reincarnation before my second child was born and then died a complete and utter exhausted death in the nineties after my second child was born .It had new lease of life age 40 after I separated from my first husband and it thrived as it had fun and realized that it wasn't dead. I allowed myself to have fun with all the clichés: the sexy foreigner, the cheeky chappie, the toy boy, the internet date and the older, rich man. My libido had some great times. I felt empowered in my early forties due to freedom and experimentation. I felt I had finally come of age.

Then I met my second husband and felt quite complete. My libido was having a lot more than fun. It had learned to connect with someone on a spiritual level. Body, mind and soul...what more could it ask for?

This continued for quite a while even though at times I was truly tired and fed up with my gynae problems. You can still have these problems and have a good sex life as long as you have a partner who is caring, undemanding and supportive. My second husband was and is. But as I headed towards menopause my libido left me, only to be replaced with tiredness, lack of confidence and self doubt. I wanted to sleep and recover enough energy for the next day. Sex was becoming a bit painful and too much like hard work. At the same time, my husband's business had succumbed to the recession and he wasn't feeling that empowered either. We were both tired, pressurised trying to keep enough income to support the family and not that content. I feel that there was an element of male menopause too and this may have been good as there was really no pressure on me to perform as such by my husband. But this, in itself, left me feeling unattractive, unappealing and sometimes quite lonely. My mind started to worry that I was the cause of our lack of sex life and that I should do something about it. But if you have no energy, it is easier to turn over and enjoy a good sleep (night sweats allowing!) Our saving grace I feel is that we were intimate in other ways. We never started the day without a kiss and cuddle and an enquiry as to how one another was feeling. We held hands during the day and were spontaneous with tickles and hugs. I don't know if we would have survived without this. When I began to count back months instead of weeks since love making, I knew I had to understand things more.

So I went back to the spiritual questions again as they had provided me with answers before for other menopausal problems. I asked myself how I felt about maturing spiritually and how becoming a wise woman was having an affect on my sex life. My husband was my true spiritual equal. Was I afraid I would move to a new level and leave him behind? I had seen spiritual inequality spell the end for many loving relationships. When a loving partner moves upwards on their spiritual path they can sometimes feel the need for new partner who matches them more. But this wasn't the case for my husband and me. I felt that he was mature in his own spirituality and had always been way ahead of me magically anyway. I felt no need for someone else and was generally happy in my marriage. Therefore, the spiritual argument wasn't working. My spiritual progress was not interfering with my sex life, it was the physical symptoms and mental anxieties that were. I still felt very connected to this man. It was simply that my libido had done a runner and therefore was compromising my spiritual sexuality. This needed a different type of meditation, a different type of solution. This time I had to focus on the physical to balance out the spiritual and not the other way round.

Meditation: for loss of libido

Crystals:
Sunstone, for energy and passion.
Citrine, for confidence and humor.

How do I really feel?
(Oh spirit. I feel an important part of me is missing. The sexual and sensual connection I am due as my human right is missing. That total intimacy, that sense of completion is no longer mine due to the changes in my body and mind. My body is letting me down, depriving me of my sacred sexuality. If I am to be a wise woman, I need this side of me to be nurtured. My egg basket may be emptying, but my soul needs tended and my relationship needs nurtured in a sacred sensual way. I miss this connection. I miss the fun of it, the laughter of it and the sheer release of it. To have found this completion, only to lose it, is too painful to contemplate. Let me learn how to manage my physical symptoms so that love making will not be a chore. Let me make the effort to find my libido and fire it up again.)

Mantra:
(My libido is only hiding. I can find her and fire her up again.
Libido... I am coming after you. I will find you and we will work
    together.)

Other ways forward:

The physical symptoms had to be brought into balance. I used the meditation described in the chapter 'chin hair, and belly hell'. I used this to build up my confidence and to empower me but it wasn't quite enough. I had to empower my libido. Imagination and visualisation seemed the next trick up my sleeve. I loved my husband but sometimes familiarity can breed contempt or in our case 'content'. I had never looked at anyone else while I was with him, but it was now time to waken things up. First step was a Daniel Craig calendar, set up in the laundry room to relieve the boredom of ironing. A famous singer once said to the husbands of his adoring female 40 something fans ' I start the engine, you drive it home' and I feel he had a good insight into female sexuality. If we don't use it, we lose it. A few James Bond movies and my libido wasn't putting up such a fight. Next was You Tube and a catch up with the videos of my favourite eighties band. Reliving how I felt as the bass guitarist strutted about the stage made me remember how good it was to lust after someone unattainable. Some good old raunchy girl talk with my sister and best friend over cocktails led to an appreciation of female desires and the humor of sex. Taking the pressure off my husband to be the person who reawakened my libido made it a personal act of empowerment. I realized I was recapturing my libido on two separate occasions. The first was my daughter's 18th birthday party when I felt the need to tell her that one of her long haired male friends was 'hot and that I wished I was thirty years younger'. Later on that week, I came back to bed in the small hours after my usual trip to the loo and noticed that my husbands' shapely bottom was poking out from under the covers. Instead of covering him up lovingly, I just had a longer look.

By focusing on the purely physical, the sense of spontaneity was coming back. I wanted to be physical again. But would my confidence hold out? Would I have the confidence to instigate sex? This was helped by another meditation; one that would focus me on the love and pleasure that could be shared by me and my husband. We were older, our bodies not as they once were. We had aches and pains and bad backs and a prolapse. I had to believe that older age and constraints would not stop our spiritual sexual link.

Meditation: for ongoing connection as a sensual couple

Crystals:

Rose quartz, for being open to love.

Sunstone, for energy and passion.

(I am becoming the wise woman, the grandmother. You are older and less vital, but we love one another all the same. We have shared intense love and I wish for that to continue. I stand before you. My breasts hang lower, my belly is bigger, but my smile lines are all for you. Our bodies are different now. I will not hide from you. This is me now, as I am. I know that you love and accept this as I do you. Let us now kiss and make our way in sacred sexuality, connecting as only we know how. Grandfather, I honor you! I am the Grandmother. We fit!)

Chapter 8

Where Did My Babies Go?

I had two babies, both girls, five years apart. In the middle I had a traumatic miscarriage. I had already established myself in my career as a pharmacist before I had my first daughter, Jennifer. I didn't have much maternity leave with her as money was tight and my first husband was showing signs of the crippling depression that would eventually kill our marriage. I needed to work, as most women did in the eighties, to manage a family, home and lifestyle. I felt I could do it and performed the usual juggling act of motherhood/career woman/wife/daughter of elderly parents. By the time Jillian came along five years later I was an old hand at this and lack of sleep was just a side effect of the way things were. I had a few more months off with maternity leave with Jill than I had with Jennifer as she was not an easy baby. I always said if I had had Jill first there wouldn't have been a number two child. When Jill was three years old I gave up my pharmacy career to follow my dream of becoming a full time clairvoyant. This again meant very hard work and sometimes a lack of time with my children. In the eighties and nineties women were encouraged to 'have it all', to follow their dreams. I was ambitious but not just for myself, for my children too. I wanted them to grow up into confident, ambitious young women and felt that the best way to do this was to show them that a women could work hard and still have a good family life. I was also scared of not having money. My husband's illness meant that he had lots of time off sick and his career was sadly affected by this. He lost jobs and I came to feel that the only way forward was for me to make sure that we were all alright. So I worked, and worked hard. My girls were my joy and I had such

43

good relationships with them, even during the terrible two's and teen's! By the time menopause hit me they were both young adults excelling at their chosen subjects and proving to themselves that hard work could bring them good outcomes in life. They were simply two of the best things in my life. Two caring, wonderful, quirky daughters who loved their mum and who were very definitely their own persons. What more could I have asked for?

I wonder if my close bond with them was what made the emotions that followed so very, very hard to manage. The feelings I had as I went further into menopause simply tore me in two. I am finding it so hard to actually write this, my hands are shaking and my tears are falling already.

I had always looked forward for them: to first days at school, to exam results, to university places. Now, to my horror, all I could do was look back. In looking back I was focusing on all the things I had missed and all the things I might have done wrong. My intellect told me I was a good mum and had always done my best. The proof was the two young women about to embark on their own adult lives in a good and exciting way. My emotions took my back to every decision that I had made along the way and found me lacking. How could I have gone back to work after just eleven weeks maternity leave with Jennifer? How could I have entrusted her to a childminder? The childminder was simply wonderful and was Jill's for a short time too. But how dare I put work first? These were my babies and I should have been at home with them! How could I have missed the first time Jennifer pulled herself up to stand at the childminder's sofa? What type of selfish mum launches a new career when her children are eight and three years old respectively? The trips to London to make a TV show were exciting for me and helped my professional profile, but were they right for my children? Did they miss me when I was away? Did their dad look after them well enough or was he slumped in front of the TV, feeding them Cheerio's? What about when I went away to spiritual retreats to learn more about spiritual development? Were these times selfish? Should I have waited until they had grown up? My head knew that when I was away my girls were well looked after by their dad and grandparents. They loved seeing their mum on TV and were proud of my achievements. They enjoyed being surrounded by my slightly bohemian friends, learned well from other cultures and spiritual paths, and didn't blink when my gay friends came to stay. They listened intently to the Native American elder who came to visit my house and were delighted when he sat chatting to their friends in his Washington Redskins cap. They enjoyed their time camping down in a tepee when their friends were going to Tenerife. It was all quite an experience and they turned out fair minded, non bigoted young women. I could see that. But my heart was pounding me to death with all the 'what if's?' The imbalance of menopause was making me question the way my life had gone and it was debilitating me.

As if this wasn't enough, I could not help the memories of when they were small coming unannounced into my head. I would be looking at one or other of them as they did something normal and practical and I would be transported to another time, many years ago when they were babies or toddlers. The memories were clear and in hard focus, like I was back there living them again: Jennifer in her red polka dot dress and hat; Jill in her tartan jumpsuit at her uncle's wedding; Jennifer at eighteen months with her first pair of 'John Lennon' spectacles; Jill with her beloved Buzz Lightyear; Jennifer as a bride at Halloween; Jill playing in her bath. Overwhelming, magical memories, all of which reduced me to tears. My babies: where had they gone? Where had the years gone? Where were my little girls, my nativity play angels, my real life dollies with imperfect ponytails? They were gone for ever, replaced by the best gift of all: two young women who were also my best friends. So what the hell were all the tears for?

It was at this stage that my girls realised that I could cry for Scotland! Nothing was off limits. I could cry when they made a joke, when they made me a coffee or while they were telling me of their exploits at parties. My elder daughter's boyfriend, Sean was part and parcel of our household by then. Sometimes I would look at him and find that I was thinking about the baby I lost and knew had been a boy. Once I even called him by my lost baby's name. I was horrified. I was mourning my girls growing up and also mourning the baby I lost. So, more tears then!

I think the emotions tied to my children were the worst part of menopause. Maybe even worse than the mood swings. Some days I just felt like I wanted to go back and relive it all again. Towards the end of my moon pause time, Jill decided that she wanted to move out to go to university. At the same time, Jennifer announced her engagement! I was so happy for both of them. Inside I was dying. I tried to convince them that my tears were of joy, not of despair.

Menopause and empty nest syndrome all at the one time! How would I cope? Was this one of my final tests in becoming a grandmother? I was facing not only the feelings of emotional separation but the real, deep anxiety of physical separation too. How could I live without these daughters? The last 24 years of my life had been about them. How could the strands that had been woven together for so long in happiness, in sadness at times, be unwoven in a harmonious and happy way? How would I survive without the rhythm of life with my daughters? I needed to start the process for me so that it wouldn't be so hard for them. I would not allow this process to be any harder for them than necessary. I didn't want their excitement or hopes to be tinged with 'what about mum?' Didn't I have a life? Didn't I have a loving husband and good friends? I would not let my love for my daughters be harmed by my dependency. I would handle this and I would handle it well.

So, the first thing I did was allow myself to cry as much as I wanted. Some days I would simply sit and let all the old memories wash over me. I looked at old photos and smiled and cried all at the one time. I talked to them about when they were babies and what they said or did. The more I did this the easier it became. I didn't fight the emotions. I didn't stop the tears. I let it all flow. I let it simply be what it was.

Something odd happened too. I started to think about my own mum more. I had studied at a university close to home and had stayed there until I left, age twenty one, on my wedding day. I closed the door that morning full of excitement and happiness for my new life. I didn't think that my mum's tears were anything more than a happy mum on her daughter's wedding day. I was the last child to leave and my parents were in their sixties. I visited regularly and was a good daughter. But not once did I consider the trauma my parents might have felt at my leaving. It just didn't cross my mind. My dad was on antidepressants for the first time in his life after I left home. I never once thought he might be missing me and the patterns in our lives. My mum never complained but she seemed anxious a lot of the time and sometimes lonely. Oh how I wished I could have gone back and been more considerate. I wanted to hug them both and tell them that I now understood. But by my menopause time, they had both passed into spirit. Hindsight is a great thing, but sometimes comes too late.

Meditation: for dealing with the memories and emotions of children growing up.

Crystals:

Apache tears, which is a special form of obsidian that legend says has the ability to allow our tears to flow when they should, unhindered and with dignity.

Smoky quartz, to soak up negativity or self absorption.

What am I really feeling?
(Oh Spirit, what am I to do? These memories of when my children were young are coming unbidden and uncontrolled into my head at all the wrong times. I can't stop crying. I doubt myself as a mother; did I do the right thing for them? Did I nurture them enough? Will they remember the good times more than the bad? Did I teach them enough about life and bad things and potential pot holes in their journeys? Why didn't I spend more time with them? Why is time spinning out of control? How can I move on knowing that all the best times as a mother may well be behind me? This is so hard. Too hard to bear at times. Help me!)

What can I do now to make me feel better?
(I can let my tears flow as they need to. I am in mourning for the past; a good past, but the past nerveless. I can flow into the memories. I can laugh at them and cry and remember them in every detail. These memories are good. I will take them forward with me and use them as a powerful reminder of how much I have lived through and achieved. I will carry them with love. I will see this as my time of memories and hold them deep in my heart with pride. I was and am a good mother!)

Mantra:
(Someone wise once said of menopause 'your egg basket is empty but your memory basket is full'. So be it! Let the memories flow!)

Menopause and empty nest syndrome all at the one can be very traumatic. On the Medicine Wheel, the emotions sit in the South. They are opposite the intellect in the North. In situations where the emotional direction is simply overwhelming, a good technique is to work on the aspect directly across the axis. So if you can't face dealing directly with emotions, then simply turn on the intellect and let it overcompensate. To intellectualize emotions, it can be good to write a list, to read a self help book or to use your intellectual knowledge of a problem and work with it in this way. It is a way of temporary distraction. When tears are near, do a crossword. When memories hit and you don't have time or energy to let them flow, make a list of jobs to do that will make you feel in control instead of drowning. When you sit in a child's room after they have moved out, let the emotions flow but when they are just too overwhelming, make a list of things that need done, cleaning, painting and buying new furnishings. Could this room be a nice home office for you? What about a spiritual bolt hole? It isn't wise to keep everything as it is. Intellectualize the emotion and then act on it!

Meditation: for empty nest syndrome

Crystals:
Hematite, for strength of purpose and white howlite for determination and will.

How am I really feeling?
(Oh Spirit, my life is changing. My role of hands on mother is coming to an end. My children are moving out and on with their lives. They have new times ahead and they are excited. I will not be so much in their heads as they enjoy their new lives. But I know I will be in their hearts. I am sad. I am worried about feeling lonely and bereft. I want to support them without being an emotional burden. The house will be empty; full of memories and full of silence. I do not know if I can cope well with this. Please help me.)

What can I do now to make me feel better?
(I can look at my life and the gaps that will be left and I can fill them with things I have wanted to do. I can write more, I can swim more; I can have more time to explore becoming older with my husband. I can reignite our passion for one another and life in general. I can write a list of all the things that are unfinished

due to lack of time. I can help my children in practical ways as their new lives begin. I can gift myself time to sit and simply think or reminisce. I can allow myself to develop my own new ways, new rituals and new desires. I can make this work for all of us. I am strong.)

Mantra:

(An empty nest deserves to be cleaned, reorganized and made ready for new little birds whether they be creative thoughts, new passions or unfulfilled dreams. I have new space. Let me fill it well!)

Chapter 9

Disaster: The Breakthrough Bleed

In loose medical terms you are through menopause if you have
had two years without a bleed if you are under 50 and one year
without a bleed if you are over 50. To be a wise woman or grandmother, it is seen as 13 moons without a bleed or thirteen cycles
or months. The time leading up to this is described as being
perimenopausal. In fact the term menopause itself is confusing
and I feel can really only be used totally in retrospect. But it is the
term we use to say that we are in the period of change that
includes lack of periods. and all the other symptoms associated
with oestrogen levels falling. Many women, including myself,
have quite major perimenopausal symptoms which they don't
really assign to anything apart from being a bit more tired or
emotional. For me it was the sweats that gave me the big clue
that something strange was happening. With other women it is a
lack of libido, vaginal dryness, skin changes or moods. These can
all hit many years or months before any real changes are seen in
the monthly flow of blood.

One of the major problems is that when you first miss a
period you are more likely to put it down to stress or 'just one of
those things. The first reaction can be to swallow hard and run to
the pharmacy for a pregnancy test! Then maybe you will have
another period a little later or a month later and all is forgotten.
It is only after you miss a few periods that a little light bulb goes
on in your head and you start to count. It can also be easier to
deceive yourself than actually own up to the fact that the wheels
of time are marching on and that we are heading into older age.
Many women will not be emotionally ready. They may feel
young and lead youthful lives and their mindset will be one

which doesn't really involve the word menopause.

I had been having sweats and some symptoms for a wee while. But when I missed a period it was after a time of terribly heavy blood loss. I was bleeding every two weeks and was exhausted. Although my doctor said he felt I was heading for menopause and that we would monitor what happened next, I thought that missing a period was more likely to be due to the fact that I had no more blood to give out. I was exhausted and felt that at some point, my system would need to balance itself. It was only after I had missed three moon flows that I started counting and thinking 'yippee this could be it'. I was suffering more and more from symptoms and had started to meditate and I was so fed up with all the gynae complications that I had had over the years, that menopause, in some ways , was to be welcomed. In all of the emotional and mental upsets that menopause was presenting me, I never once actually mourned not having the cramps and heavy bleeds, or the bloating or the fortune spent on sanitary protection. It was deeper and more about the changes that were happening to me on a spiritual and emotional level. By the third or fourth month without a bleed I was actually becoming more up beat about the freedom that not bleeding was giving me. I could swim whenever I wanted to without worrying that I would have an embarrassing accident. Gone were the days of astronomical bills for sanitary protection that needed changing every two hours.So although I was sad about many other aspects, the lack of bleed side of it was suiting me well.

By my ninth missed period I was hopeful that the end was in sight. Only four more months to go and I could be judged to be through menopause and also adopt the role of grandmother if that was what was to be. That worried me a bit too though as I didn't feel nearly there at all spiritually. I had developed meditations and was trying hard to adjust to my new sprit name but to be honest, I felt a bit premature. I worried that when the time came for me to accept the grandmother role that I wouldn't be ready for it spiritually. Certain rituals I had planned to do had not come about either because of hiccups or delays. Sometimes the weather got in the way; sometimes the moon sister I wanted to come with me wasn't able to come. I really didn't feel as though I was on the right schedule spiritually.

Then it happened: the breakthrough bleed. Right at the new moon of my tenth month without a bleed. I had felt cramps and had been very tired. I had put the previous days of irritability and sadness down to menopausal symptoms. Instead I had had fierce PMT but not recognised it. The bleed was bright and red and there was no confusing what it was...a period! It only lasted a couple of days. Even as write this I can almost taste the despair I felt. To have come this far only to backtrack seemed unfair and downright wrong! I was angry...the Creator must have been a man to play such a cruel joke! No women would ever do this! The Universe was stopping me in my tracks, delaying my plans, forcing me to start counting again. Couldn't I just ignore it? What could I say to those who were now interested in my progress and spiritual development? I was so annoyed at myself and my body and dreaded the thought that this might just be the start of many further bleeds. I went to bed, cried, punched my pillow and felt very sorry for myself indeed. I couldn't even think about what it meant spiritually. I felt a fraud.

I told my closest moon sister and asked for her to send healing as she was excellent with distant healing through Reiki. She immediately started to tune in and sent warmth and healing. She told me that in her healing she still sensed all the grandmother energies in me and that this was just a temporary delay. I felt a bit better for this and decided to meditate and see if I could find some answers. A break through bleed is not unknown in the menopausal journey. (Always check with your doctor if you have any unusual symptoms with it and if it happens after you are deemed to be through menopause. Bleeding that is at all unusual should be carefully examined) But spiritually it seemed like a major crisis to me.

I took myself off to a quiet restful place. My family and husband knew what had happened and were very supportive. On this occasion I decided just to see what would come and what answer may unfold. Whatever I learned could be incorporated into a new meditation later. I took myself and my bruised ego into deep trance meditation by dancing and swaying until I felt my hips would break. I remember crying and wanting to know exactly what Spirit's plan was for me. I waited for my guide to come but when he did come he was silent. I asked him to fill me in on what was going on. I was so angry! In his own way, he answered enigmatically, 'You know already. You told the Universe what you needed.' I understood. Although I had been coping reasonably well with the physical and emotional changes, I had been feeling overwhelmed by the rush towards the spiritual outcome. I had felt as though it was all galloping forward too fast. I had wondered if I would have had enough time to learn all that I felt I needed to be the grandmother I wanted to be. I had needed a sabbatical, a break, a time to realign, to gather my thoughts and to be more in the moment. The Universe had listened. Great Spirit had given me what I asked for...more time! I knew instinctively that it was right and felt a surge of clarity and deep connection, of thankfulness for being gifted time to prepare more, time to assimilate what I had already learned. With this in mind, it felt right to start counting again. I knew that this breakthrough bleed would be a one off and that instead of fretting over the coming spiritual responsibility I now had another thirteen moons to prepare and to be all that I could be! It made sense and I welcomed the intervention.

The following meditation is to help acknowledge and accept the breakthrough bleed for what it is: a pause, a slowing down, a time for reflection of what has gone before.

Meditation: to cope with the breakthrough bleed

Crystals:

Moonstone, to help balance out menstrual patterns.

Bloodstone, to help release the blood flow and correct blood imbalances and sodalite, to help define the truth of the matter and give emotional clarity.

What I am truly feeling?

(Aho Great Spirit. Today I am in despair. Today I am shocked and have been knocked off balance. After nine months, enough time to conceive and carry a baby, you have given me back my moon flow. It is hard to understand. I felt I was doing so well. Maybe my ego needed grounding? Maybe I was becoming complacent in my spiritual progress? Or maybe it was just as it should be? I needed more time and you have gifted me that. So why does it still feel like a step backwards? Can you help me go back and count again towards my thirteen moons without moon flow? Can you help me to work with this delay and show me all the further things I need to know? Can you reassure me that this moon is all part of your plan? Spirit, help me to know more. Help me to learn more. Help me to understand that this delay is for my benefit to help me be the best grandmother I can be.)

Mantra:

(I subconsciously pushed the 'pause' button: Spirit has responded! I wished myself more time: Spirit agreed! How wonderful!)

Chapter 10

The Panic Attacks

In my teens I was an organised student, a practical workhorse who studied and coped with older parents and their health issues. In my twenties I was a professional pharmacist and pursued my career with self belief and ambition. In my thirties I juggled children, husband, home, bereavement of my elderly parents and changes to my career. In my forties I became more spiritual and enjoyed the calm feelings that this brought to me. I have always been a list maker, a Taurus who liked plans and security but I have never really been a panicker! So, in the lead up to menopause, I was completely over whelmed by my first panic attack. I actually didn't know what it was and thought I was going to faint or, even worse, die!

I was in a very busy supermarket and I was pushing my laden trolley around in a crowd of Saturday morning shoppers. I had done this hundreds of times before. I cannot think of anything that was so extraordinary about it. The crowds were pushing and the aisles were very busy. I think I remember being bumped by another trolley and feeling pain at the back of my ankle. My first reaction was just to move out of the way but the shoppers all seemed to want to be in that one aisle at that moment and there was no where to move to. In the next few minutes, I thought I was dying. My heart began to beat wildly, I started to sweat and yet I felt cold and clammy. Was this a heart attack? Was I going to die in a supermarket with none of my family around for last succour? Other shoppers were pushing in on me and I felt like shouting but my mouth was completely dry and no sound would come out. I held on to my trolley for dear life and leaned in towards the cool dairy shelf hoping the air flow would revive me. The atmosphere seemed charged with anxiety and chaos…yet everyone else seemed to be going about their business unaware of these energies. I was finding it hard to breathe and was even more panicked by the thought of having an asthma attack with no one close to help me. My ears were buzzing and I felt I was going to keel over into the dairy cabinet. As I struggled to breathe and felt myself becoming more and more faint, a kind woman asked if I was alright. She was looking at me as though she understood somehow. This seemed to break the chain of physical symptoms and I began to breathe easier and felt my heart rate calm down. Thank you to that woman! I abandoned my trolley and headed out to my car where I promptly burst into tears. What the hell was all that about? And would it happen again? It was a panic attack and yes, it would happen again. There never seemed to be a pattern though. The panics could come on when I was in a family situation at home or when I was shopping or on an evening out. They never seemed to come when I was working though and I instinctively knew that my pre work meditations must help in some way. One of the main causes seemed to be parking my car! I hated trying to park on a busy road in town and eventually would only park in a quiet place or where there was lots of space. Being watched by strangers as I tried to manoeuvre my car into a space made me not only have a panic attack but also left me feeling stupid and incompetent. So, I avoided parking on street. Then I began to avoid supermarkets at busy times. This evolved into shopping for groceries via the internet and having them delivered, which actually saved me money as well as energy! However, I didn't want to avoid all situations and to be honest, sometimes the panic attacks were so random that I would have needed to stay in bed all day just to avoid one. If a car was too close behind me or tailgating me, I would feel the panic start. Sometimes, if I thought about the work I had to do that day, the panic would start. If I thought about my daughter leaving home, my heart would start its crescendo of beats. If I was in a room full of people, if every one was talking at once, I would feel the anxiety build up. Anxiety was the cause mainly but at other times there seemed to be no rhyme or reason. So what could I do to prevent these horrible panic attacks becoming a way of life while I was menopausal?

The answer to me seemed linked with the fact that they never hit me during my clairvoyant readings so the meditations I did before my work must, in some way, prevent them. Was it the prayers I said or the familiarity of the pathways that were now ingrained in me as I prepared for opening up my awareness? Or was it just the fact that meditation itself is known to help calm and bring a placid feeling? I decided to try a more general meditation just for gentle calming and peaceful feelings. It wasn't aimed at any defined outcome apart from maybe giving me the general sense of peace that would stave off panic attacks. It worked amazingly well and I call it my 'Sacred Space meditation'.

Sacred Space meditation

Find yourself somewhere comfortable to sit or lie (this can be done before you get up in the morning if you set your alarm clock 20 minutes early). Surround yourself with warmth and comfort, maybe some pillows and a comfy blanket. Close your eyes and say a wee prayer that the meditation will calm you and also give you any insights that you may need for the day ahead.

Now think of a place that you associate with feelings of extreme calm and serenity. It could be a place from your last holiday or simply a place that you have felt secure. It is better if it is outside in nature and not a crowded place. My sacred space is a loch that I used to visit in the Highlands of Scotland with my family and sometimes on my own. It is tranquil, very beautiful and holds so many happy memories for me. You will have someplace like this that resonates with you and will be your sacred space. Now you have to travel there in your mind. Close the door on your house and either go in your car or walk to it or fly away in an aeroplane. Make the journey pleasant as you feel the weight of worry fall away as you become excited about visiting your special place. As you arrive at your destination, stand and look at what you see. Your memory should serve you well and you will remember a special tree or the way the water looks or how the grass blows in the wind. Take in the view and breathe out and in deeply as you enjoy the vista. Now, in your head, go and sit where you would have the best outlook and can see but not be seen. This is your sacred space. No one can come into it unless you invite them. You can view things but will not be interrupted unless you want to be interrupted.

Let your gaze take you around your sacred space and see and feel what is there. What season is it? Is the wind high or low? Is the sun shining? Can you feel the earth below you and the sky above you? What do you feel? Are you sad or happy or stressed and worn out? If you have negative energy, ask the earth to take it from you. Feel it draining out of your body into the good mother earth. Or walk in the water and let the water soothe your ills. Let any negativity flow out of you.

At this point you may be drawn back into memories of why this place feels good for you. I sometimes 'see' my dad and my little spaniel walking along the loch shore and it cheers me up as this reminds me of happy times when they both walked this earth with me. Sometimes something will catch your vision; a bird may fly across your gaze or a fish may jump in the water. Enjoy whatever shows itself to you. And yet again, release what you need to release. Or simply enjoy the view. While your mind focuses on the view, you will be subconsciously relaxing and meditating without too much effort on your part.

After 15 minutes or so, or as long as it takes, start your journey back to your starting point. Stand up, say some thanks, wave goodbye to anyone you encountered and then get back in the car/ plane etc and make your way home, building up energy for the day ahead. When you feel yourself back in your bed or chair, let your conscious mind take over and bring you back to reality. Open your eyes and move your muscles and stretch and say hello to the new day! Have a drink of water handy and make sure you eat before you go about your day's business as meditation can sometimes leave you a bit disorientated and water and food grounds you.

If you don't have an active imagination, you may have to practice more than someone who is good with visualisation. Persevere! It will be worth it and the more you do it, it will become habit and your sacred space will be accessible to you more quickly and more dramatically. I can conjure up my sacred space within a second now if I need an instant 'calm fix'.

You don't need any crystals specifically for this meditation but I find that amethyst can be good for bringing a calm feeling and also tigers eye can help you 'view' your sacred space in a more vibrant and real way. If you are worried that you may stay in the meditation, then hold a grounding crystal like obsidian in your hand. Make it a ragged one or one which isn't tumbled and let it make its presence felt to bring your back to your conscious mind. I quite like an obsidian arrow head...it can certainly make its presence felt by gently digging itself into your palm! I wouldn't recommend an alarm clock being set unless it is very unobtrusive and low. Programming soothing , gentle music can help bring you back down to earth too...but it must be measured and almost sneak up on you. Use this sacred space meditation whenever you feel the need to calm down or take control back.

Chapter 11

Angry and Irritable

I have never really been an angry person. My family is Scots Irish extraction and could have its moments but my mum never liked anger and in a way, anger may have been internalized in my family. My mum liked calm and was a bit too posh for displays of anger or tantrums. So I think I was from a brooding family where resentment built up and exploded rarely but intensely. It mattered what the neighbours heard and my parents were old fashioned and kept a lot to themselves. By the time I was in my teenage years they were in their sixties and were mellowed and secure. My first husband was volatile and his family were noisy and confrontational and it took me a long time to become used to that. I don't like confrontation and will always try to reason with someone before I let myself be open to anger or shows of temper. So, most of the time I would have been described as placid of nature and calm. It was only every so often when I saw red that folk would run for cover and again it would be more to do with sarcasm than shouting.

It was quite a surprise to me when the hormonal changes of menopause left me feeling angry and irritable at both small and large incidents. It horrified me the way I could go from calm to red hot temper in seconds and I am sure my loved ones resented the change in me. Things that in the past had registered as an annoyance became reasons to let loose and to assert my opinion. The mess in my utility room drove me mad each day but as soon as it was tidy my girls seemed to fill it up again with washing and ironing. Were they incapable of taking their clothes upstairs? If a client was late I could feel annoyance building up and had to calm myself before they came through the door. The thing was, I often started a bit late myself due to over running in readings. My rural broadband could have me raging at my PC and it in turn would react as though to stick its tongue out at me and freeze or lose my files. My cat seemed to be the most unobliging, moaning cat in the world (she was probably menopausal too!). Shop assistants who were surly or didn't know how to do their jobs left me incandescent with rage. A newspaper article on child abuse could have me scheming as to how I could do damage to the perpetrators. My poor, laid back husband was just too laid back. I wanted things done in my time and not anyone else's. I simply needed to feel in control of life and when this didn't happen, the result was anger. This was alien to me and I felt overwhelmed by this new emotion and the intensity in which it was presenting itself.

In the middle of my menopause something happened that made me feel even more out of control and ungrounded. My husband's business failed, and this, added to step family logistics and negative interactions resulted in us separating. I didn't want this to happen but whatever I did to try to sort things out simply failed. Events had happened that there was no way that I could help or resolve and I felt emotionally drained and so very, very upset. I was totally angry that once again, it looked like I had a failed marriage. I was angry at life and the universe for throwing me all this pain when I least could deal with it. I became very withdrawn and sad but had to carry on working and being a parent. I spent long hours searching for answers and when they didn't come I became angry and so very annoyed at life. I knew that it would take quite a lot of help from Spirit to help me through this.

In one meditation I had a major breakthrough. I understood in every fibre of my being that I really had no control over the situation or its outcome. I was hopeful that my husband and I would be able to mend the hurts that had separated us, but so much of that was down to him to work through his own issues.

I couldn't help. We were both on our own journeys now with all our own pain and desolation. I had hope but no real idea of what would happen. My daughters were so supportive but they had their own issues with it and were suffering because I, who had always seemed so strong, was falling to pieces. The understanding that I had no control was frightening but I knew what I had to do. My next ritual would have to be one to give up all my control to Spirit and to simply accept that whatever was right for me would come forth. I felt strangely calm as I thought on this. All my plans, all my hopes could be simply wrong. What if I wasn't meant to be married? What if I was meant to be alone? Wasn't that all right as long as it was the right thing for me? And for my husband? And what if financially we went into meltdown? I would do what I had done before and find another way. If I couldn't afford my house, then there must be somewhere else I was meant to be. Simple! I needed to let the universe know that I would accept whatever it brought to me; that harmony would come out of chaos, without my meddling or anger.

The ritual I prepared was intense and special and was helped along by synergy and 'coincidences'. I have had a connection with the Hindu goddess Lakshmi and found her to be very benevolent to me. So I decided that I would ask her to be my conduit to the universe in my intent for it to recognise my acceptance of its plan for me. I prepared my offerings and prayers to her. However, as time went by in my preparation I felt she wanted me to connect with another deity. It came about that this was Durga, her mother. The ritual of acceptance would involve that I accepted the outcomes for both myself and my daughters, that I would be strong enough for them too. Durga has two daughters and this seemed apt. So I changed my intent to be connected with Durga. This felt right but I asked for confirmation. As I was about to close my offering pouch, I felt the need to go into my spare room which I had cleaned earlier.

Lying dead on the floor was a queen bee. She hadn't been there earlier and the windows and doors had been shut. So I took her and added her to my offering pouch and only then did it feel complete. My ritual and intent and mantra to Durga are personal and between her and me, but I did ask for her to let the higher beings know that I would accept whatever outcome manifested. The weight lifted from my shoulders and I cried till I could cry no more. I buried the offering in a plant pot and planted seeds on top that were of a healing plant. Then I waited. My trust had come back and I knew myself and my girls would be fine. I felt a release from anger and despair for the first time in weeks. It was like almost being reborn. Over the next few weeks I worked when I could but spent the rest of the time focusing on the intent and on the changes that were happening. My financial situation stabilized. My health stabilised. My girls and I became closer than we had ever been. My husband worked his way through his own problems and we decided to work on being together again. After doing the ritual I felt empowered to simply trust that I would be all right. It was an amazing feeling. After that I chose to try to let feelings of lack of control wash over me. They no longer made me angry or caused me to react in such a frightened way. Six months later, the ceramic planter broke in a sudden frost. Nothing remained of the queen bee or of anything else, including metal, in my pouch. All gone. I later read that Durga manifested as a queen bee or a swarm of bees and in this way vanquished her enemies or anyone who threatened her children or family members. Thank you Durga! Thank you queen bee!

Meditation: for anger and feeling out of control

Crystals:

Smoky quartz, for sucking in anger, and aquamarine, to trust in the flow of life.

How am I really feeling now?
(Oh spirit, I am angry at the way my life is going. I am angry at little things and big things, people and animals and the universe. I don't do anger well. It upsets me. I don't know how to disperse it or if that is even the best way to deal with it. I am troubled by my temper and I can't deal with the way the anger gives me a sore head. I feel that this truly isn't part of who I am. It feels external, like a demon who takes over my thoughts. I am not an angry person but I do know that feeling out of control makes me angry. So need your help to let go of needing to be in control. I need to let go of being the person who directs the traffic and let others deal with their own issues and in their own time. Help me Spirit. I am low and I am sad.)

What can I do to help myself now?
(I can know that I am a good person. The angry me is just a reaction to feeling that everything is running away from me. I can hand over responsibility to others for their wellbeing or decisions. I cannot control what others do or their opinions or prevent their mistakes. All I can do is deal with my own problems and trust that the outcome will be all right and what is necessary. I can allow myself to be angry for a short time and work on why I am angry. Then I can let it go.)

Mantra:
(I trust in the universe to provide me with what I need.
Trust kills frustration and kills anger.)

Chapter 12

Exhaustion

Menopause can bring bad sleep patterns due to night sweats, worry and anxiety. Sometimes, sleep will just not come at all and the hours meander by while frustration builds. Sometimes sleep will come just before you have to get up and face a busy day. This can leave you feeling exhausted, irritable and totally worn out.

I had never had real problems dropping off to sleep but had a habit of wakening at about 4am and not being able to fall back to sleep. When menopause hit, I still had the 4am starts but I found that it could take up to two hours to fall asleep. Some nights I was only having about 3 hours sleep and even these were uncomfortable and fidgety. I had always been an early bird and liked to have a lot of work done by midday. As the sleep patterns changed I found myself becoming more of a night owl but without the energy to accomplish work or tasks. This, in turn, made me feel unconfident and unfocused.

Even when I slept, there was still a terrible underlying feeling of not being rested. It almost felt like when I had two small children and worked as a pharmacist and did the ironing and housework at 1am and then had to be back up at six am to start it all over again. The difference now was that I didn't have youth on my side and I didn't seem to have any reserves. The exhaustion sometimes marred happy occasions and I would be the one at a party on a Saturday night willing the time on so that I could go to bed and simply rest. If I was working at night, I needed a nap in the afternoon but, still, sometimes would sit down to work at night yawning my head off. I simply had no energy. One time I went away for few days holiday with my husband with high hopes of a romantic and fun time, only to crash out on the bed for most of the days and nights! Once again, my understanding husband didn't complain. He said he was glad to see me resting for once! I still felt bad.

I began to avoid socialising because I felt that I wasn't much fun and I didn't look very good. Travel became another drainer of energy so I restricted my 'away days' and worked more from home. Sometimes even an afternoon at the cinema with my daughter left me yearning for a nap. The exhaustion that came with menopause was one of the most debilitating things I had to deal with. I needed a practical plan as well as an empowerment meditation that would bring some energy to me.

So I started to have a nap every afternoon. Just an hour, and if I didn't sleep, I would use the time in meditation. Some days I felt worse but most of the time, the short rest invigorated me and let my intellect flow again.

I also gave myself permission just to sit still, doing nothing or reading a good book. If the weather was good I would sit outside and simply enjoy the sun's rays beating down on me. I needed time and by gifting myself this time, I felt better and coped with life in a more optimistic way. Make sure you rest. Put your feet up and simply enjoy time to yourself.

Meditation: for energy
Crystals:
Clear quartz which acts like a battery for you and sunstone to harness sun energy.

How am really feeling now?
(Oh Spirit, I am so, so tired. My body, mind and soul seem drained of energy and I feel like lead. I have no spark and no feelings of enlivenment. My body is letting me down. It needs too much sleep but it also doesn't give me quality of sleep. I am so tired and I am beginning to step away from people and social situations just to try to reclaim my energy. This may be what is

needed but the down side is that I miss my friends and the fun we have when socialising. My skin looks grey and tired out and my eyes are red and gritty. I want to have my old energy back. I need to find access to the energy source that is the sun and that will share his grandfather rays with me and give me my spark back.)

What can I do just now to help me?
(I can allow myself to rest when I need it even if it is not sleeping. I can cat nap and I can simply sit still. I can carry my clear quartz crystal with me and use it like a battery. I can carry my sunstone and feel it reflect the sun's energy at me. I can go easy on myself. I can take time out from friends and social occasions if I truly need to but sometimes must be social so that I can bask in the energy of laughter and friendship. I can sit in the sun. I can allow myself time to recharge my batteries. I can do things that replenish my energy. Things that I love doing like baking or listening to music. I can believe that this tiredness will pass.)

Mantra:
(Grandfather Sun. I need your energy!
Grandfather Sun, bless me with vitality!)

Chapter 13

Mummy's Little Helpers

In the nineteen fifties and sixties many women going through menopause were seen as hysterical and were often prescribed tranquilisers e.g. Mummy's little helpers .(This phrase was coined, I believe in a song by the Rolling Stones in 1967 to describe the widespread use of tranquilisers among women.) Many women became prescription medicine addicts as a result of this. Although these medicines had a place for women who truly needed them, they were widespread in use and could cause side effects of lethargy and emotional dullness and of course, addiction.

The other extreme of menopause can be seen in Jane Austen's Mrs Bennet in Pride and Prejudice, full of the vapours and mental exhaustion, relying on 'taking to her bed' and annoying the life out of her daughters. I felt there had to be a way of handling menopause symptoms without relying on medication OR retiring to bed for 3 years.

I had decided to make my menopause as simple as possible and was interested in seeing how I could manage it without anything unnatural in my system. I also decided to avoid taking any herbal medicines. When I was a fully practising pharmacist I recommended herbal medicines and was happy to do so. However, it is wrong to assume that natural means non toxic or safe. Some herbal remedies are extreme in action and some can even be fatal if the dose is exceeded. They can also have quite unpleasant side effects. Plus, some have claims associated with them that are not that accurate. I feel that these medicines should be prescribed by a fully qualified herbalist or pharmacist unless they are proven, traditional herbs and from a reputable source. Even then, I feel an herbalist will know more about the nuances of them and their interactions and should be consulted. So, for my menopause I decided to try and avoid all prescribed medicines, even herbal. This was my choice, and may not be yours. I wanted to see what would happen if I really just went with the flow and worked with the meditations and mantras I loved so much. If I added a medicine to the mix, even an herbal one, how would I know what was helping? This didn't mean that I didn't have my own 'little helpers'. Certain things helped certain aspects of menopause more than others. Here is my list:

Smudging with sacred herbs

Smudging is a technique where certain herbs are set alight, blown out to release their smoke and then wafted either through your aura to cleanse and rejuvenate it or in a place to improve its energies. Smoke, from herbs and incenses, is used in many cultures for this. The easiest way to do this is to buy a smudge stick that has the plant dried and tied for you already. You need a strong flame resistant dish or tray or abalone shell. Light the stick and then blow on it to dampen down the flame and release the smoke. Place it in the dish. If you are cleansing your aura, sit the dish in front of you and with cupped hands or a feather, waft it to either side of your head, then above. Push the smoke through your aura gently and do this several times. You do not need to breathe in the smoke.

My favourite plants are used in Native American rituals and both cleanse and bring positivity. First use sage, either Californian White or Mexican. It is like strong spiritual disinfectant and will push out negative thoughts, energies and emotions. It can sometimes leave the aura depleted and with 'gaps' though, so it is wise to follow this with sweetgrass. Sweetgrass brings positive, happy energy and can make you feel absolute joy and harmony almost as soon as it is used. While smudging with these herbs I use the mantra 'Cleanse, Bless and

Protect'. Smudging once a week or more can help you maintain a sense of balance and hopefulness. It is so good if you need to let go of angry emotions and despair. Always make sure the smudge stick is fully extinguished as they can burn from the inside out and can be very dangerous if left unattended. Also avoid lighting one directly under a smoke detector!

For smudging a room, e.g. after an argument, start at the door and waft the smoke all the way around the room in a clockwise direction, returning to the door and sealing the room in sacred smoke. Again, take care not to burn yourself or carpets by not wafting too vigorously. This is where feather or feather fan can come in far handier than your hands. Other herbs that I have found useful are lavender for its calming properties and cedar to aid grounding when you feel a bit out of it and disorientated.

Asthmatics should be very careful and take advice from a doctor as any smoke can aggravate the condition. Always be sure you are not pregnant (some women assume they are menopausal when their periods stop, when they might just be pregnant!)

Aromas

During menopause I found that my sense of smell changed and very much for the better! Aromas seemed more intense and so much more evocative. I found that certain perfumes from my twenties became firm favourites again and that scents gave me exquisite pleasure. It wasn't just perfume though, the smell of freshly baked bread or coffee being filtered made me feel cosy and happy. Lighting a scented candle provided me with away to be transported to a warm beach, a forest, a lemon grove or a winter wonderland of pine and Christmas scents. My house had to smell good or I didn't feel good. My nose was hyper sensitive and any whiff of cat food or rancid food could make me physically sick. On the other hand, lavender could soothe me to sleep; rose geranium could make me strangely joyful and frankincense, quite serene and spiritual. If you feel your sense of smell becoming more intense, why not use this gift as something to help you too, in your new life journey?

Chanting, music and dance

Silence can be good but also oppressive. I have always loved music and it can change my mood within seconds. Often a piece of music from the past has brought instant happy or sad memories. Music connects us to moments. It weaves through our personal history and can be like a marker to events in our lives. It connects us to people and how we feel about relationships, past and present. A Christmas carol, a lullaby, a song a parent used to love, the song of our first love affair, the song that played on the radio when someone died and has stayed melded to that moment...all examples of how music can influence us.

I used music like a therapy during my menopause. I knew it could change my mood or encourage me to really submerge myself in memories that were necessary for my healing. I don't feel we should apologise if we feel miserable and I honestly feel it is better to embrace the moment for a while rather than ignore it. When I was so sad after my first marriage failed I chose to listen to Toni Braxton's 'Unbreak My Heart' when I felt low. It made me cry, helped me to release the tears and I felt better after it. Sounds mad? No! Crying releases endorphins that lift our mood, so there is science to back this up. In menopause I felt the need for uplifting music, music that made me want to dance. Much to my husband's annoyance Lady Gaga became my new uplift. I needed to be able to stomp about and move. I had no energy but couldn't sit still if some dance music came on. At parties I danced till my knees hurt. It was like being a teenager again.

Dancing has always been a passion of mine. I did contemporary dance and in the eighties did dance movement, jazz and in a mad moment also tried to learn to tap. As menopause hit I felt my joints stiffening and my muscle tone declining. I swam, which helped but it didn't give me the thrill of simply moving to music. Putting a CD on in my kitchen and boogying away lifted my spirits and gave me a bit of exercise and made me feel younger ...until my knees hurt the next day! Why not try to have a wee dance in private to lift your spirits? Or go the whole hog and join a salsa class?

I learned to chant at some Native American gatherings. I had no confidence in my voice but eventually joined with others to chant some basic but enjoyable chants. Since then I have learned more but have only about five that I use regularly in certain situations. One is a power chant that can really build up energy and allow me to focus on the task at hand, whatever that may be. Another is a beautiful lullaby which I find restful. Another is a birthing chant which helps when feeling crampy or moonish. You could listen to some indigenous chants and see what you connect with? Or you could simply sing your own mantras? It may feel odd at first but it can be powerful to release your voice.

Homemaking

When was younger and busy with career and raising small children, I didn't have time to worry too much about being house-proud. I preferred my children to feel they could be creative even if that meant a messy living room or toy strewn garden. I relied on ready meals at times and didn't own a spice rack. There was simply no time for the indulgence of elaborate meals or pristine carpets. As my girls grew older I became more interested in cooking and making my home look nice. To be honest, my home was clean but not that tidy. Any spare time was spent learning new spiritual ideas or honing my tarot skills.

Menopause didn't change me into a Stepford Wife, if that's where you think this is going. No! Comfort always won over beauty. As a Taurus, I liked lovely things but I wasn't that materialistic and wasn't that bothered if ornaments were broken by kids or wallpaper showed signs of wear and tear. In the course of my menopause, I felt a surge of creativity where homemaking was concerned. I learned how to make things and actually enjoyed making them. My favourite thing became cooking a huge Sunday roast dinner and feeding anyone who wanted fed. I nurtured through food. I learned to bake and asked for a birthday present of a bread maker. The house smelled of fresh bread and home baking and I enjoyed making meals from scratch. There were a few disasters but on the whole, I was pleasantly surprised and pleased at my efforts. I made limoncello liqueur for Christmas presents and searched antique fairs for pretty bottles for it. I became obsessed with old embroidered table cloths and flowers. I grew my own herbs and even dried flowers for pot pourri. I looked for ways to reuse just about everything and planned treats in advance so that I would have time to make them very special. 'EBay' and 'vintage' became my new worlds. Quality mattered and the older the better. I found a simpler, more enjoyable way of being a home maker. This seemed to soothe me and make me feel more feminine and grandmotherly. If you feel the urge to make jam or learn to knit or anything else that seems at odds to who you were, why not give it a go? You might find, like me, that it becomes a genuinely enjoyable way to relax and to feel connected to family and friends.

Creativity

My creativity had always flowed through writing. Whether as a teenager, new mother or as part of my work I had always written and enjoyed keeping journals and puting my thoughts into words on paper. I had written a psychic agony aunt column for a syndicated newspaper for years and had been a tabloid astrologer. I simply adored writing but never had the time for more than short stories or writing courses based on the tarot or shamanism. My short stories were normally humorous and I wrote pieces for friends sometimes just to cheer them up.

As I progressed through menopause initially, I felt the need to write more so I began to keep a menopause journal but sometimes I just felt that my creativity was blocked. I wasn't that confident in my writing.

Then Spirit gave me a reason to push through the lack of confidence. A friend of a friend was looking for new authors of spiritual material with a view to publishing and asked to see my work on the tarot. It was accepted but I had to rewrite it so that it flowed more as a book rather than a tutorial course. Could I do this? What would it involve? Wasn't I already too busy? I thought about it for all of three seconds and decided to go ahead with it. Wasn't this what I had always dreamed of? And what a gift from spirit at a time of turmoil. It was something just for me. Synergy was also at play, as it would mean hard work with writing and promotion just at the time that my younger daughter was planning to leave home for university. What a wonderful distraction! Once my first book was finished, my proposal for this one was accepted and I felt on top of the world. Letting my creativity out in writing has been a saviour to me in this time of change. It has brought much happiness and confirmed my initial beliefs that menopause was meant to be a time of positive motion not stagnant energies.

What have you done in the past that was creative that you maybe lost the connection with due to either lack of time or confidence? Poetry? Writing? Drawing? Calligraphy? Or do you just feel that maybe it is time to see if you actually do have a creative side? Then, take my advice and just say 'yes' to exploring it!

Massage, cuddles and kisses
Touch is important. It makes us feel cosy and loved. My daughters seemed to know when I needed an extra cuddle or a great big hug. Sometimes that was all I needed to help me stop crying or to give me the courage to walk out the door to a business meeting or event. They would sit either side of me and

squash in while we watched a TV show, or would stroke my head when I was sitting stressed out at my computer. Little touches and shows of affection could lift me up and keep me going.

My husband would massage my neck when I had a headache or rub my back when I was tense. He stroked my forehead and face at night if I couldn't sleep and gently soothed away worry lines. At times he scratched my back when I was being driven mad with a menopausal itch. I have always been a tactile person and these touches had always been there, but they became more important as menopause progressed and I felt more and more insecure. Kisses are sweeter when you really do need them. Whether it is a kiss from a partner, child or friend, don't rebuff it. You need all the help you can get! If your partner is a bit unemotional or not confident in showing feelings, this can be the time for you to educate him on your needs and reward him so that these new ways can become new patterns that will see you through the difficulties and problems of old age. Use menopause to change old patterns of connection.

Demand what you need if you have to. Human beings need touch: menopausal women need it even more!

New image

I am naturally red headed, a Celtic ginger! I am over weight and prone to looking pale and washed out. Before my menopause, I wasn't really that unhappy with my body as it did what it said on the tin as such. It was a good vehicle, it carried me about, it had been strong and it had given me two lovely children. So what if I had stretch marks, wrinkles and hair that was described as 'in a bad mood' by my daughter! I was happy to be alive and kicking, I had found new love and remarried in my forties and generally was too busy to worry about my appearance that much. I made an effort to be groomed for my job but was equally happy with no make up and my hair tied back at weekends. I liked fashion and girly things. My style, if it could be called that, was groomed bohemian!

During menopause things started to change and I became a wee bit more experimental. My shape changed and not in a good way, but if anything I became more flamboyant and more 'in your face'. I dyed my hair baby blonde...so much easier on the root retouch problem. Red heads tend to go a kind of steely grey and this was no good for my complexion. The new blonde proved a hit with my husband and daughters and I felt younger and lighter. I was so happy with it. My hair had always been a tangle of curls and my daughter straightened it for me. From curly red to straight blonde was such a transformation and I loved it! I did it for no one but ME and that, in itself, felt good. What else was there to experiment with? Sparkly nail polish? No problem and lots of fun. Leggings? The madder the print the better! Maxi dresses? Great for covering puffy ankles. Eyeliner? Can you get away with that when you are older? Yes and add some metallic eye shadow just for effect.

I think that subconsciously I was aware I was becoming invisible as a menopausal woman, no longer being looked at in a sexual capacity. This in itself was liberating as it meant that any changes I made were definitely only for my benefit. I became bolder with prints and patterns, handbags and shoes. Fabric texture and comfort became necessities as did natural fabrics to help battle the hot flushes. As my menopause progressed I accrued a new image. Bigger, bolder and more flamboyant. I was refusing to be ignored, marginalised or drained of personality just because I was becoming older. I preferred the new 'me'. It sat better with who I was and I was now only dressing for me. I had no 'uniform' whether that be for work or play. I was just enjoying being a newer version of myself with no one but myself to please. Why not try it? Let a new image be one of the things that punctuates your menopause; one that you are comfortable with but one that also reflects who you are, what is going on in your life and to hell with the consequences!

Nature

The power of connecting with nature is that it can make you feel very little, very humble and very unimportant in the grand scale of things. Personal worries melt away when the sun beats down on your bare arms. Big insecurities seem small when the stormy waves come crashing onto the seashore. Resting your back on a mighty tree trunk can dissolve feelings of self importance or self absorption. Feeling a cold river rush around your ankles can invigorate and take puffiness away. Nature is there to take us out of ourselves and to let us see the true flow of things. Women's lives are like the seasons: we have our own rhythms. Menopause is one of them. So let nature inspire you, humble you and take you out of yourself!

During my menopause I found I yearned to be close to water. Anything would do...a river, the seaside, a stream, even a garden pond! Water soothed me and cleansed me just by its ebb and flow, its reflections and its incandescence. I also found that wilderness inspired me and made me feel like I belonged to something bigger, vaster than my own little life. I holidayed in a very remote cottage in the Scottish Highlands and the solitude and magnificence truly lifted my spirits. I saw eagles and hawks, butterflies and bees, deer and hares. And lots of sheep! I saw animals nurture their young, birds hunt for their food and bats enjoy their evening swoops. In all of it, I felt connected and special, without being that important.

I also made a point of exploring my rural area. There were many local beauty spots that needed a bit of extra time to reach or were hidden away. I gave myself time to wander and simply relax in my own company. Connecting with nature helped me breathe, helped me off load anxiety and made me stronger by allowing me to connect with natural rhythms and the beauty which is our earth.

Chapter 14

Moon Sisters

The Importance of Women

As my journey into moonpause waddled on I became more and more aware of the need for women in my life. I have always had many male friends and enjoyed their friendships which in some ways were less complicated than with women. The majority of my clients were women, but only a few of my close friends. My mum had passed into spirit many years ago and my birth sister had her own life and we weren't close. My best friend and comrade lived 150 miles away and although we met up regularly and used the internet every day, it never felt like enough. I didn't have a mum, or granny or aunties to lean on for support. My daughters were supportive, my best friends but they were young and I didn't want to burden them.

A few years previously I had hosted a moonlodge, a monthly meeting of spiritual woman who gathered at the new moon to honor our paths and womanhood. It was something I looked forward to and it allowed me to experience different ways and different rituals. We meditated and prayed and discussed our problems and then we ate chocolate and had a laugh. But this moonlodge had been disbanded as we went into new jobs, new areas or new directions. We still kept in touch but not that regularly.

I missed having my spiritual time with women. It made me think of the way things were in ancient times or in tribal societies where women were nourished and respected and where the feminine was seen as a force for good.

In ancient civilisations, when women lived closely together, they menstruated at the one time, at the new moon. They went to a place to honor their moontime and to look after one another. This was a time of relaxation, of community, of passing on of knowledge and of giving the powerful moon blood to the earth. In some Native American societies, this is called a moonlodge and was a tipi or structure reserved for this process. The young girls cooked and brought food and they and the women of moonpause looked after the men and the normal day to day activity of the tribe. The moon sisters could eat well, burn sacred herbs and deal with any pain or discomfort. It was a magical time and was honored. After 3 or 4 days, the women would come out rejuvenated and ready to move towards the full moon, when they would ovulate and maybe conceive. So the moonlodge was a time of letting go of last month's blood and stress and the time spent with women formed bonds and connections that would help in times of trauma. In our modern societies we just keep going through moontime, we do the same amount of work, we don't really give ourselves space and we really don't allow for it to be a spiritual time of reconnection with ourselves. So we don't renew, we don't feel our strength and magic, and we are all the worse for it. We get PMT. We run on empty. And by not claiming our space, I feel that the whole idea of moontime becomes devalued and glossed over. We think of it in negative terms e.g. the curse! We don't allow our men to see that we need time to go with the flow as such and either be alone, have time away from the kids or simply explore our magic. This makes us less as women and we need to teach our daughters a new way of upholding these old ways. Moontime is not an illness but it is a time that needs to be accommodated and made to be the best it can be.

I remember my first moontime. I was eleven. My mum handed over the 'talk' to my older sister who showed me how to put a sanitary towel on and that was it really. A few months after the 'talk', when I did start to flow, I thought I was dying. And after that this bad thing, my period, just stopped me swimming and doing the sports that I wanted. I wasn't allowed to wash my hair for some reason and it was all treated like an embarrassment. Yet, in tribal societies a girl's first moon is celebrated and the tribe sees it as the start of her fertility and increasing the fertility of the tribe. Rituals can take up to four days and there are gifts and initiations and the young women are made to feel very special indeed. So unlike my first moon/period and those of women my age. With both my daughters, I gave them presents and made them feel special. My friend's daughter asked me to be her moonmother. This is the person who the young girl nominates to look after her during her time after her first moon and who will help and guide her in life. It is an honor to have this role. I hope my daughters follow in the old traditions made new, so that their daughters may benefit from an awareness of how special their moontime is.

And then there is our way of looking at moonpause. There are two extremes: either that it is an illness to be fought with every medication/procedure or it is something you just get on with. Both points of view miss the point. To treat moonpause as an illness and medicate against it robs you of your right to be a grandmother, a wise women. But so does ignoring it and just getting on with it. This means that you are not considering it as a special time at all. You will miss the nuances and the delights, the illuminations and insights that only time concentrating on your journey will bring. An older friend of my daughter asked her how I was finding 'my special time'. I was taken aback by the phrase...but yet, she is right, it is a very special time. I wouldn't miss it for the world.

Again, in tribal societies a woman heading for moonpause is seen as special. She is coming into her time where her blood no longer flows out to create life, she holds it within. From within it can become her new creativity, her passion, her wisdom. She can use her blood for the greater community now, not just to reproduce. Her insights become greater, her advice more well thought out, her sense of the bigger picture more intense. She is respected and her opinions valued. In our current society, this does not seem to be the case. Women at moonpause become invisible unless they take on the characteristics of males. An older woman is seen as less attractive in her natural state. This is helped along by those who fight moonpause every step of the way, trying to outsmart nature and remain youthful with toxins in their forehead and silicone fillers keeping their old breasts suspended like a 20 year olds. How sad! Yet each to their own. I believe that nature will always win and at some point she will show us the lack of wisdom in filling your body with things that your immune system sees as a threat. I believe that if you constantly try to trick your immune system, eventually it will give up trying; leaving you with no defence system for when something really does need to be fought.

I do accept that this moonpause wisdom etc may not be for everyone: there are always going to be silly old women just like there are silly young women. I believe, though, that it should be our right to have that wisdom if we want it and not to live in a society that values youth above anything else.

In looking at the older ways or ways of tribal societies, I saw that women seemed to be nurtured at the important stages in their life and I missed the fact that my generation has somehow lost that.

It was time to reconnect with women in all stages of life. I had nicknamed my best friend and spirit sister 'Cloudy'. My nickname was 'Stormy'. Stormy and Cloudy go well together. We are anamcara, soul friends. With her help, we started to chart my moonpause and to prepare for a final ceremony and to learn from my experiences not only for her when her time came, but for our daughters and their daughters. We made time for ritual and we explored old ways of doing things. I learned to make bread, she learned to weave. We danced in the North Sea much to the delight of onlookers who were wrapped up against the cold. The water was frozen but we didn't care: we did it because we could! We took time to do 'sister' things physically and spiritually. For every birthday or special occasion, we invented a cocktail. If we didn't have the information to do a ritual, we made it up ourselves. This strong sister connection helped me in every way. It made me feel supported and loved and understood.

I also reconnected with female friends from the past. Some of this was done through social networking, some by chance meetings, although I don't believe it was chance. I began to surround myself with women of all ages and walks of life. My daughters became more involved in my moonpause and offered support and much love. I may not have had the tribal structure of the past, but I had as close to it as I could in this modern world.

Meditation: to bring female friendship and support
Crystals:
Moonstone to connect with the true power of the feminine and pink quartz to have an open heart.

How am I really feeling now?
(Oh Spirit, where are my female friends and family as I go towards my moonpause time? Have I been guilty of letting my friendships fizzle out when they have become a burden? Have I taken the easier option of more straightforward friendships with men? I miss close female friendships. I miss my mum. I miss the family structure of a time gone by. I need to be closer to the feminine and to enjoy friendships with women of all ages. Please bring me the connections that will allow me to feel nurtured and supported. Please allow me the strength and confidence to say yes to new friendships without looking for an agenda. Let me support women and let them feel nurtured and cared for by me. Let females come into my life and let me enjoy feminine pursuits and feminine humor. I need to be able to trust women and to learn from them again.)

What can I do to make me feel better now?
(I can try to reignite old friendships that I have let fizzle out through lack of time or energy. I can understand that females of all ages can support me as I go towards moonpause, not just other menopausal women. I can be open and warm and encourage these connections with a soft word and an open ear. I can be empowered by the women I already know and in doing so, in some way, empower them.)

Mantra:
(I welcome my new female friends, sisters of the moon.
I deserve these friendships and I will honor them when they come.)

Chapter 15

The Magic of Moon Pause

In many books on spirituality we see the triple energies of the goddess i.e. maiden, mother and crone. As I have said before, my own spiritual path calls the crone energy 'Grandmother'. It is my belief that many patriartrical societies and religions have turned the essence of the crone into something to be feared, something ugly to be hidden. The aspect of the virgin or mother is seen as more acceptable and not quite as scarily powerful as the woman who holds her blood within and is responsible for great vision and prophesy. So much of the magic of the grandmother has been lost as oral tradition has been lost and so much of the remaining spiritual or religious writing has been done by men who were clerics of patriarchal religions. The power of the post menopausal woman was in some ways made either frightening or comical. Children were told to go to sleep or the Banshee would get them; Snow White was offered the apple of death by the warty, craggy old witch. The post moon pause woman reminded people of death. After menopause we are nearer death and if we can be ignored then we do not remind others of that sure fire ending. If we cannot be ignored, then at least let us be either satirized as something of terror or made into comical creatures to be derided. In this way, the crone has been marginalized and because of this there are not many books to be found on the magic of this important time for women. I could find very little at all and found that talking to moon pause women and clients helped me more than trawling the internet.

I wanted to know how to take the magic I had learned from being a maiden and then mother with me into my grandmother years. I knew it would be different but I didn't feel that all that went before was irrelevant. I was right.

During my moon pause, I still sometimes 'felt' my old moon flow even though it wasn't there. I had a sense of fullness and the occasional wee cramp. This is described as 'moon memory' and had been felt in different ways by my older moon lodge women. In one it was still quite a powerful feeling even after 6 years of no longer having a moon. In one it was almost like the unexplainable tickle you get when a baby stirs on the womb. In another it was an agitated state. These women could have continued to use this energy when doing magical ritual but all chose instead to use the stronger and more accessible cycle of the moon in the sky.

In ancient tribal societies most women came together and menstruated at the new moon and then could conceive at the full moon when ovulation took place. I was lucky: my moon memory was at the time of the new moon anyway. So I could use both the new moon and my own moon memory if I wanted to express myself through ritual at this time. At some point my moon memory may cease but I will be happy using sister moon for her energy and cycles. So, the magic or intents or prayers that you may have done while menstruating can still be done. Just do them at the new or dark of the moon. Those that you may have done while ovulating, just do at the full moon and watch the magic work! As a moon pause woman you can now be aligned totally and amazingly to the moon herself and work and learn from her cycles of power.

It can also be good to continue to use moonstone crystals to align you with the moon now rather than your own past menstrual cycles. Moonstone is especially powerful when used in intent at the full moon. It embodies the ultimate feminine, the goddess energies.

The grandmother or wise woman has lived and breathed and seen happiness and sorrow. Part of her magic is a greater under-standing of this in others. As such those of you who have healing magic can expect it to be empowered after moon pause. There will be an opening of compassion and empathy like you have never known and it can help with feeling what is wrong with a person and therefore in helping to put it right. You may find that you see auras for the first time or that you access your spirit guide more easily. Where before you struggled with visions and maybe could not understand your dreams, you may find that you have a new found clarity.

Also with the compassion and the clarity and healing, there will be an inner sense of confidence and also sheer determination. You may not tolerate fools gladly. You may find that silliness and shallowness make your inner crone mad as hell. That is when the Banshee will come out wailing! When Kali Ma will shake her skulls at the people who will not listen to her: When Durga will turn herself into a queen bee and sting those who try to hurt her offspring: when that Grandmother who is you will pick up her medicine shield to protect the tribe.

This may also be the time that you feel you have outgrown your name or your past identity. It might be time to ask for a new name or a new animal totem or spirit ally. If this is meant to be, then it will happen. My new name of 'Sunfire' sits quite well with me now. My main totem or power ally of mountain lion is still so relevant but I feel very close to birds now especially hawks and falcons. So magically I am the same but different; still me but more so!

You will not loose your magic unless it is meant to be shed for something greater or more YOU! Don't fight this process if this is happening to you; trust that the universe will not let you down. I have seen post moon pause women go from Wicca to Christianity and vice versa, and some go from clairvoyance to healer and vice versa. Some have even moved away from ritual magic to become political and use their new strength directly to hit at the male dominated hierarchies. Think of being you but more so!

Chapter 16

The Role of the Grandmother
and the Grandmother Ceremony

If you look at ancient or tribal societies, the post moon pause woman had a special role. She was not necessarily the leader of the tribe or most important elder. She was seen as having her own wisdom and her own domain of power. When she was younger, in moon flow time, her blood was there to nurture and bring life to the unborn child. She was the nurturer, the women who held the fertility of the tribe. After moon pause, the blood no longer flows and is said to be kept within. This internalising of the blood flow can then be used as a fire for creativity, for new passions and also for the nurturing of the whole tribe, rather than just the children. The post moon pause woman is seen to be a powerful holder of knowledge and a person who can be relied upon to have opinions on larger life issues. Basically, she knows the score! Her vision is freed from the day to day tasks of looking after the young and can therefore be more panoramic. The grandmother can be the advisor to the younger women, holder of the traditions and be a respected guide to the men who seek out her wisdom. She will not be good at everything but will have her own talent or sphere of knowledge that she will excel at. She will take on her role with dignity and with patience. She will still be learning and honing her skills. She will expect to be both listened to and looked after.

How different is this to our own modern societies, some of which see an older woman as a burden or a waste of space? How far have we come from Great Spirit's teachings that we let someone old and wise sit in their own excrement in an under funded nursing home? How far have we travelled away from tribal respect when a child can call an older woman derogatory names and swear at her? My heart is sad with these thoughts.

Only we can change this by instilling goodness and manners in our younger generation. But we have to aspire to that respect and show society that we have worth and deserve our place in this world, both in advisory roles and leadership roles. If our children and grandchildren see us raging against the aging process by filling our faces with botox and our breasts with silicone, what message does that give them about the dignity of ageing? Why deny our wrinkles? Are they not the signs that we have lived and have the knowledge of life and happiness and sorrows? If a grandchild cannot depend on her grandmother for advice and love because the grandmother is not interested in her own little tribe, then what type of grandmother will the child go on to be herself? Where will the links with the past be? The links to family traditions? The family stories that make us feel part of a clan; make us feel we have roots and that we belong? It is our responsibility to make this time of our life relevant; to make older women relevant. We will not be unheard if we walk our talk with dignity and the expectation of being heard.

My gift as a grandmother is my vision, my clairvoyance. I will use it to help those who ask for help. I will use it for the bigger picture too. By this I mean that any feelings of earth changes or visions of future society that unsettle me will be noted and talked about. I will not be silent. I have already journeyed and seen the future regarding chaos and trauma in certain areas of the world. These have been documented and passed on to those who can maybe help to change things. My other gifts are compassion and unconscious humour. What is your gift? You may not know yet as you may still be on your journey, going through your rite of passage. It will come. It may be something intense like a new interest in politics or society. You may become connected to a charity or a cause. Or you may simply be the kindest, most loving person your family know. You may develop an all consuming interest or passion and will learn about it and pass it on. Or you may decide to live on a croft and live in harmony with nature. Let your moon pause show you the way for YOU.

A grandmother can be cosy and warm and dizzy and wise. She may have a harsh tongue when it is needed. She might be all things at one time but she should never be ignored. Stand in your own power! Yes, it is your time but it is also your time to influence society and to be heard. Your blood held within can give you the confidence to speak out and the knowledge to right many wrongs. Spiritually this is what a grandmother does. Her focus is now not only on her own children but on ALL children, on society and on the very growth of love. With integrity and wisdom she can give the understandings that can heal feuds. She can show the way by living her beliefs. She will be a standard bearer for what is expected in a caring society. With this great responsibility will come much love and much pride. Let us take the role of the grandmother back and put it in its rightful place in society. Only then will older women gain the respect and dignity they deserve.

My experience of moon pause has been intensely personal and amazingly intense. As my 13 moon cycles without a bleed draw to a conclusion I can think on what I have learned and also begin to prepare for my grandmother ceremony. I have learned a lot about myself, my strengths and weaknesses, my fears and heartaches. I have lived each moment with intensity and, at times, have felt wounded by these emotions. I know that wounds heal, that emotions are transitory in nature and that time really does bring healing. I know that I am strong and can rely on my own strengths to do anything I want in life. I know that Spirit is present in every decision I make and in every connection that comes my way. I have found my true creativity and have my passion back. I have learned that it is all right to cry, to weep rivers. This is cleansing.

I have also learned that the true feminine is present in every age of woman; that moon pause is just part of this, no greater, no less. I have learned to appreciate my life and count my blessings and I am a calmer and more compassionate person. I am also more prone to say exactly what I feel or mean even if it comes over a wee bit sharp at times.

I have learned that life holds simple pleasures: a comfy bed, a real fire, companionship and mirth, a child's smile, a letter from an old friend. These simpler pleasures mean more to me now. I appreciate life as something amazing and as something to be cherished by truly living it, not rushing about, not being materialistic. It is a time in life to enjoy friendships and family and, if possible, a contented relationship.

I do not have the energy I once did for truly physical pursuits. My knees don't work well and I have to curtail the physical pleasures that once were so much part of my being. It would not be sensible for me to ice skate again because of my knees. But I can remember when I ice skated with sheer joy and abandon and the memory of doing it is enough. Memories are like presents from the past that nurture us into the future. I adore sitting and simply reliving lovely times. Memories also stimulate creativity. You can learn from a memory about what you once felt passionate about and go forward to recreate it. You can also learn how to act or not to act from a memory. As your memory basket becomes fuller, your wisdom will become more all encompassing. You will access the past, present and future all at once. This is the place of the grandmother: a place of no spiritual limits!

Grandmother Ceremony

So, now it is time to plan my Grandmother Ceremony. I am sure there will be little things that are so personal to me that will just fall into place when they are needed. I will let my daughters and moon sisters know what I would like and they will help. In fact, the planning and carrying out of practical tasks will be mostly theirs. This will leave me time and space for reflection on my new responsibilities and new role. There are a few traditions that seem right and time honoured. Yet I feel there will also be new ones which we bring forth ourselves. I look forward to seeing what these will be and how we will implement them.

The day will be chosen not only to suit myself but to suit others too. This will be my first gift to my family. No one will be left out and no one will be without a place.

There will be a shawl that will represent my stepping into the grandmother role. This will be a focus in the ceremony. Family and friends will be asked to give something of theirs that can be sewn onto the shawl as a lasting sign of physical connection and emotional links. This can be a little feather, a special symbol of the person, a poem, or a piece of embroidery or anything that seems appropriate. It will be well thought out and will allow me to connect with them in the future, even if they are far away. It will have their essence in it and will help me to connect with them in my healing role of grandmother.

There will first be a cleansing sweat lodge for myself and any females who wish to take part. This will be my time to cleanse and prepare for the spiritual part of the ceremony. Although the grandmother ceremony is female only, my husband and spirit brothers will be asked to participate by being fire keepers and stone carriers for the sweat lodge. They will stand guard as warriors outside while we women cleanse through prayers and chants.

After the sweat lodge I will be prepared for my ceremony by my closest moon sister and my moon daughters. This will involve anything from helping me dress to helping me do my hair. I will be me, simply and honestly…so I will want my make up on and my mascara! While this is being done, the place of ceremony will be prepared by other females who will make a circle out of flowers and rocks and have special symbolic plants in the four directions of the Medicine Wheel. This will be an honoring of my devotion to the Medicine Wheel as well as my ceremony. It will be in itself a teaching for those who follow.

Each direction will be held by one of my two daughters and my two close nieces. They will have thought about which direction they will hold and will understand what that direction means for someone who is becoming a grandmother. On this occasion I will enter the circle from the east direction and will l walk clockwise round all four directions, pausing at the west. There I will walk over the symbolic bridge between south west and northwest, symbolizing my walk into the new life pattern. Then I will move to the centre and the moon daughters will tell me of their directions, what they mean to me and their hopes for me. I will then say what it means to me to be a grandmother and make my pledge to my extended family to be the best grand-mother I can be. My closest moon sister Cloudy will approach me and I will hand her my personal moonstone. This will symbolize handing the moon to her as she then takes on the role of mother to the family. She will then bring the shawl and lay it on my shoulders. I imagine I will be in tears by then.

The circle will then be exited to be closed down by Cloudy who will then indicate that the ceremony is closed and the party can begin! I will have music and chants and drumming. There will be wonderful food and lots of laughter, hugs and kisses and much talking. Anyone who wishes to give a gift will be able to at that point. Gifts can be little mementos like poems or candles. As the party goes on I will do my 'giveaways'. Giveaways are little gifts that thank the people who have helped with the prepara-tions. They can be as simple as a candle or some home made jam. Wine will flow, music and dance will follow and no doubt I will collapse into bed feeling every bit my age!

I have been lucky enough to be invited to a grandmother ceremony before and this was the general flow of it. It was one of the most emotional and happy ceremonies of a rite of passage I have ever experienced. Thank you to Looking Elk for the invite.

This ceremony is quite elaborate and will be time consuming.

You may prefer a simpler ceremony and it may only have you and a few girlfriends attending. Make sure that you honor this personal rite of passage in your own way. My ceremony may give you some ideas, but think about your life and what you would like. Would you maybe like to do a fire walk with your sisters? Or how about a night under the stars? Or a day at a health spa followed by a ceremony in a local beauty spot? The choice is yours and will only be meaningful if you do what really is in your heart. This should be a marking of the end end of your 'special time', the beginning of your new wisdom and new way of living. The life you lead now may be very much the same as before but it will be lived with a sense of contentment and harmony. Or it may be totally different as you embark on all the things you have wanted to do but never had the time. Whatever the result of your moon pause, let it be a time of happiness and connection with Spirit. Walk in beauty, balance and harmony!

Acknowledgements

Thank you to everyone at John Hunt publishing and O-books who helped me along the path of writing and releasing my creativity.

Thank you to my doctor and staff at Blackwood Surgery for being compassionate, professional and then leaving it up to me!

A big thanks to my spirit family and friends especially Malcolm for just being Malcolm! And Sooz for being there for me...all the time!

To my beautiful daughters: I hope this book helps you in years to come and I thank you for your understanding of why I needed to write it. Thank you for your support.

And a big thank you to Jim, my husband, who was the main recipient of my moon pause madness! If you can survive that, you can survive anything, my darling! Thanks also to Sean for help with diagrams.

Thank you too to the women of Silver Birch Moon lodge and to the family of Standing Trees Medicine Lodge, I have learned so much from you all.

Thank you, Icamna. Thank you to my clients both male and female who inspire me with their courage and strength when life throws them trauma. You all do not know how strong you are!

**AYNI
BOOKS**

Ayni Books publishes complementary and alternative approaches to health, healing and well-being, following a holistic model.